ASTHMA

●Ayurvedic Cure ●Herbal Remedies ●Yoga & Meditation

Dr. Anil Mehta, Dr. R.N. Sharma
Dr. N.K. Gupta

Special Feature
SARS

HEALTH ❦ HARMONY
An imprint of
B. Jain Publishers (P) Ltd.
An ISO 9001 : 2000 Certified Company

> **Note from the Publishers**
>
> *Any information given in this book is not intended to be taken as a replacement for medical advice. Any person with a condition requiring medical attention should consult a qualified practitioner or therapeutist.*

ASTHMA: AYURVEDIC CURE, HERBAL REMEDIES, YOGA & MEDITATION

Edition: 2003

Reprint Edition: 2007

All rights are reserved. No part of this book may be reproduced, stored in a retrieval system or transmitted, in any form or by any means, mechanical, photocopying, recording or otherwise, without any prior written permission of the Author.

© Copyright with Dr. A.K. Mehta

Published by Kuldeep Jain for

HEALTH 🌳 HARMONY

an imprint of

B. Jain Publishers (P) Ltd.

1921, Street No. 10, Chuna Mandi,
Paharganj, New Delhi 110 055 (INDIA)
Phones: 2358 0800, 2358 1100, 2358 1300, 2358 3100
Fax: 011-2358 0471   *Email:* bjain@vsnl.com
Website: www.bjainbooks.com

Printed in India by
Akash Press, New Delhi-110 020

BOOK CODE / ISBN: 978-81-319-0193-9

RREFACE

मनः प्रसादः सौम्यत्वं मौनमात्मविनिग्रहः ।
भावसंशुद्धिरित्येतत्तपो मानसमुच्यते ।।

भागवद् गीता 17/16

'Manah-prasadah' means purity and the mind is free from morbidities, like cheerfulness of mind. In other words, when dejection and fear, anxiety and grief, agony and perturbation etc., is filled with light and vivacity, it is said to be cheerful.

Complete absence of such afflicting morbidities as coldness, jealousy, violence, vindictiveness, ferocity, ruthlessness etc. and the constant placidity and coolness of the mind is known as 'Saumyatvam'.

'Maunam' means the constant application of the mind to the thought of the virtues, glory, truth, essential character, sports and names etc., of God or to an enquiry about Bramah or the Absolute.

When the restlessness of the mind totally disappears and it gets steady and thoroughly disciplined, it is said to be controlled. This is what is known as 'Atmavinigrahah'.

Bhavasamsuddhi means the complete elimination from the mind of evil propensities like partiality and prejudice, lust and anger, greed and infatuation, arrogance and malice, jealousy and animosity, scorn and contumely, envy and intolerance, obstinate error and idle thought, aversion to what is desirable and contemplating what is unwelcome on the one hand, and the constant blossoming of virtues like forbearance, love, politeness etc., on the other.

All the virtues mentioned in this verses are connected with the mind, and eradicating all its impurities purifies it; hence they have been spoken of as the austerity of the mind.

Knowledge about herbs as remedies originated thousands of years ago in various medical disciplines of the world, especially in India and is generally recognised that Ayurveda, the traditional system of medicine of India, which has been preventing succour to the suffering humanity for more than three thousand years is a repository of medical experience and knowledge about well-tried herbal drugs.

Widespread prevalence of asthma is one of the undesirable consequences of modern civilization. In modern system of medicine asthma is considered as on ailment, which is very difficult to cure. This is not so in Ayurveda.

Day to day activities of an individual affect most of the organs of the body. For this reason, Ayurvedic physician always emphasize on good conduct, behaviour, regimen, etc. along with the intake of proper diet and medicine.

AUTHORS

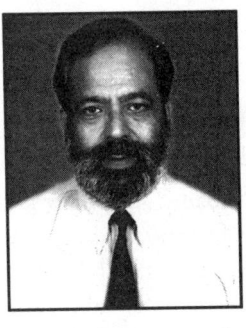

Dr. Anil K. Mehta was born on July 6th, 1954 in Jalandhar City of Punjab in a family of Vaidyas. He did his graduation in Ayurvedic Medicine and Surgery in 1977 from the renowned Maharishi Dayanand University, Rohtak in the north Indian state of Haryana and was busy in practicing Ayurveda till 1980 in New Delhi. In the year 1980, he went to Holland and is practicing Ayurveda as a consultant Physician specializing in Panchakarma. He is the founder Chairman & Medical Director of European Institute of Scientific Research on Ayurveda EISRA and has authored many books on Ayurveda and Panchkarma in English, Hindi & Dutch languages.

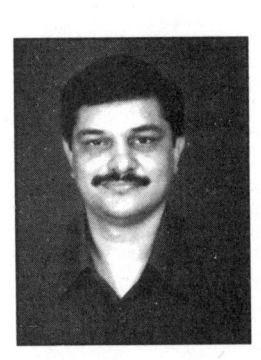

Dr. Raghunandan Sharma was born on January 9th, 1966 in Amritsar, Punjab in a family of beaurocrats and graduated in Ayurvedic Medicine and Surgery from the University of Delhi in 1990 and did his post graduation, M.D. in Ayurveda from the renowned Ayurvedic University of Gujarat, Jam Nagar. He did his thesis on Kaumarbhritya (Paediatrics) in 1993 and is a visiting Prof. & Fellow to EISRA, Holland, Turkey and Germany. He was a Research officer with the Ministry of Health & F.W., Govt. of India, and a Medical Supervisor in one of the WHO projects. At present he is doing research on Environmental Hazards on Paediatrics ailments as his Ph. D. topic. He also guides to Ayurvedic research scholars and is working on several projects related to challenging diseases. He is also consultant to many natural herbal cosmetic industries.

Dr. Naveen K. Gupta was born on August 30th, 1960 in old Delhi in a family of academicians. He did his graduation with honours and distinctions in Internal Medicine, Surgery, Pharmacology and Gynaecology from the prestigious University of Delhi in 1983. He did his post-graduate course in rehabilitation techniques in 1986 from All India Institute of Physical Medicine & Rehabilitation from Mumbai under the Ministry of Health, Govt. of India. He is a visiting faculty and fellow to EISRA, Holland. Dr. Gupta had attended several international seminars on holistic approach of medicine in India and abroad. Dr. Gupta is a recipient of Prof. S.N.T.M Foundation Award for outstanding contribution in the field of Ayurveda. He is an active office bearer on the committee for international affairs to All India Ayurvedic Congress, India.

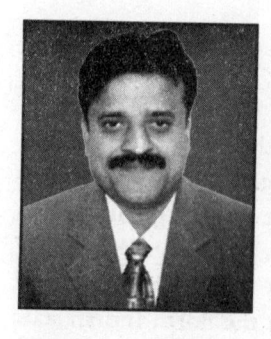

Dr. A.K. Mehta
Dr. R.N. Sharma
Dr. N.K. Gupta

Contact Addresses
Ayurvedisch Gezondheidscentrum Nederland
Thijssestraat 16, 2521-ZL Den Haag
The Netherlands
Tel.: 0031-70-3192546;   Fax: 0031-70-4140818
Email: info@agn-ayurveda.com
Website: www.agn-ayurveda.com.

Ayurveda India
H-38, South Extension, Part-I
New Delhi - 110 049 (India)
Tel.: 0091-11-24641132;   Fax: 0091-11-24648034
Email: ayur@ayurplanet.com.;   Website: www.ayurplanet.com.

Ayurveda World Wide
12, Shakti Vihar, Pitampura,
Delhi - 110 034 (India)
Tel.: 0091-11-27011148;   Email: ayur@ayurvedaindia.org.
Website: www.ayurvedaindia.org.

CONTENTS

1. **Introduction (9 to 28)**
   - Anatomy of the respiratory system 10
   - Physiology of the respiratory system 13

2. **Main diseases of the respiratory system (29-36)**
   - Hypreventilation syndrome 29
   - Rhinitis (pinasa) 31
   - Influenza (pratishyaya) 32
   - Tonsillitis (kanthashaluk and tundikeri) 33
   - Bronchitis (shwasnalika shotha) 34
   - Bronchiectasis (shwasnalika prasara) 34
   - Pneumonia (shwasnak jwara) 35
   - Tuberculosis (rajyakshma) 35

3. **Asthma (37 to 70)**
   - Occurrence 39
   - The human and economic burden 39
   - Epidemiological evidence 39
   - Childhood onset asthma 40
   - Adult onset asthma 40
   - Embryology 41
   - Who are prone to asthma 43
   - Nature of Asthma 43
   - Chain reaction leading to asthma 48
   - Effect of allergens on asthma 49
   - Cosmetics and asthma 50
   - Role of pollutants 50
   - Causes of asthma 52
   - Provoking factors 54
   - Histopathology 55
   - How does asthma develop? 57
   - Asthma and skin diseases 63
   - Season and asthma 63
   - Pregancy and asthma 64
   - Types of asthma 64
   - Consquence of sleep in respiratory muscles 65
   - Diagnosis 66
   - Grading scale of dyspnoea 68
   - Management 69

4. **Ayurveda concept (71 to 94)**
   - The tridosha concept 72
   - Natural urges 77
   - The concept of sapta dhatu 79
   - Mala 80
   - Srotas 80
   - The concept of srotas 81
   - Concept of agni 82
   - Concept of ama 83

- General causes of asthma 83
- Vyadhi (disease) type 84
- Types of asthma 84
- Concept of dosha-dhatu-mala concept 85
- Pathology of asthma (samprati) 87
- Avran 88
- Signs and symptoms of asthma 91
- Prognosis of asthma 93
- Home rules for asthma families 93
- Wrong practices in day-to-day life 94

5. Preventive measures for asthma (95-109)
- Avoidance of causative factors of asthma 96
- Avoidance of over-eating 96
- Avoidance of cold drinks and sour juices 96
- Avoidance of tobacco 97
- Adverse effects of tea and coffee 97
- Prevention of constipation 97
- Avoidance of suppression on natural urges 98
- Anxicty, desire, tension and asthma 99
- Beneficial fruits, vegetables and Beverages 100
- Food and Rules for eating in asthma 101
- Harmful effects of curd (yoghurt) on asthmatics 103
- Control of weight 103
- Avoidance of excessive use of drugs 104
- Use of preventive drugs 104
- General Tips of the prevention of asthma 107
- Regulation of daily and seasonal routines 108

6. Role of yoga in asthma (111-122)
- Yogic therapy for asthma 112
- The nose: A pranic biodetector 115
- Yogic breathing, total breathing 117
- Scientific Yogic lifestyle 122

7. Curative treatment (123 to 133)
- Management 123

8. Herbal treatment (135 to 162)
- The herbal approach 135
- Anti asthmatic herbs 136

9. Things to be observed (163-166)
- Cough and asthma 163
- Sputum and asthma 163

10. SARS (167-178)
- Severe acute respiratory syndrome 167

* **Glossary of terms** 179-182
* **Abbreviations** 183-184
* **Bibliography** 185-186
* **Index** 187-195

1

INTRODUCTION

During the past decade, despite an increasing understanding of the pathogenesis of asthma, there has been an alarming increase in the morbidity and mortality due to asthma. These days, we do a great deal of injustice to the lungs and the entire respiratory system. Our dietary habits are not sound. We indulge in excessive quantities of tea, coffee, alcohol and tobacco in the form of cigarettes, fast food and fried food. Dust and pollution, add to the problem. We are addicted to narcotics and intoxicating drugs. All these factors, including late night dinners, meetings, parties, tension, pictures, etc. are likely to affect the functioning of the lungs.

Modern sciences, with many discoveries to its credits, have, at the same time, driven man — both his mind and body — away from nature. Instead of going to religious places for meditation, he prefers to go to clubs which is not bad, but we must take care of giving proper rest and relaxation to body and mind at least for 1 hour per day when we are awake.

People who look apparently healthy begin to show symptoms of asthma and bronchitis all of a sudden because of exposure to cold, wind, rain, dietetic irregularities, mental strains etc. Asthma can be caused by affliction of the lung, heart, liver, kidneys, brain or any other organ or system of the body. Many chemical and synthetic remedies have been developed by modern medical science to prevent and cure asthma. These drugs provide only temporary symptomatic relief and their continuous use not only proved to be ineffective but also produced serious side effects.

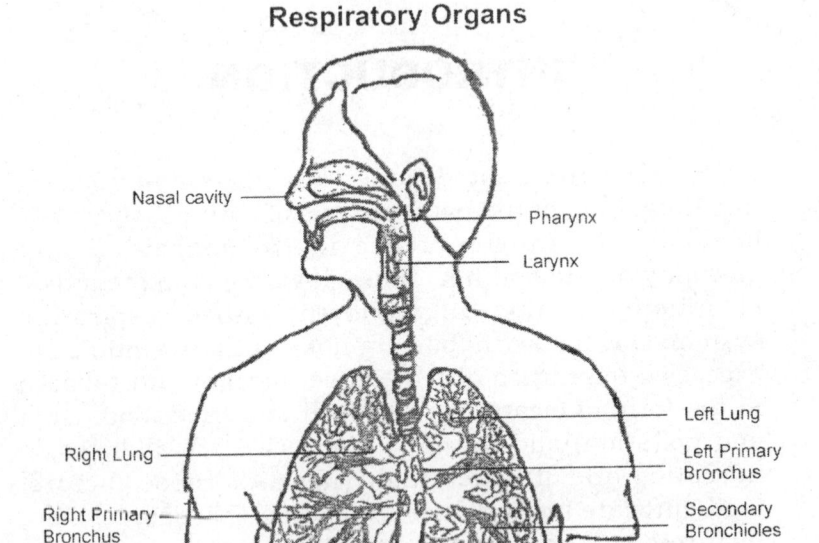

Respiratory Organs

Labels: Nasal cavity, Pharynx, Larynx, Right Lung, Left Lung, Right Primary Bronchus, Left Primary Bronchus, Secondary Bronchioles, Tertiary Bronchioles

ANATOMY OF THE RESPIRATORY SYSTEM

The respiratory passage includes the nasal cavities, nasal pharynx, mouth, oral pharynx, larynx, trachea and the lungs. The mouth and pharynx have a dual function; they serve as parts of both the respiratory and the alimentary systems. When air is passing through the pharynx, the opening between pharynx and larynx remains open but when food is passing through the pharynx, the opening into the larynx is closed. The larynx is a specialized portion of the air passage, containing the vocal cords, and in addition to its respiratory function it is also concerned with voice production. Gaseous interchanges take place between the blood and the inspired air in the lungs.

Nasla Cavity

The nasal cavity is divided into right and left halves by a median septum, which extends from the nostrils in front to the posterior nasal apertures. The walls of the cavity are composed mainly of bone and cartilage. The mucous membrane of the nasal cavity gets a rich blood supply, which permits rapid warming and moistening of the dry inspired air. It is pink or red in colour. The Paranasal sinuses are air-containing spaces communicating with the nasal cavity and lined by a mucous membrane. There are four sinuses on each side: (1) Frontal (2) Maxillary (3) Ethmoidal and (4) Sphenoidal. They vary in both shape and size. The Paranasal sinuses (P.N.S.) are small at birth, but increase in size with the growth of skull.

Nasla Pharynx

The nasal cavity communicates with the nasal pharynx via the conchae. These are oval in shape, being about 2.5 cm high and 1.25 cm wide. It is separated by the free posterior edge of the nasal septum. Pharyngeal tonsil is a collection of diffuse lymphoid tissues situated deep in the mucous membrane of the root and posterior wall of the nasal pharynx. The tonsils are well developed in childhood, and if they are abnormally large, they may block the conchae and interfere with nasal breathing.

Larynx

The larynx consists of a number of cartilages articulating with one another and connected by muscular, fibrous and elastic tissues. At its upper end, the larynx is connected to the hyoid bone and at its lower end to the trachea. The larynx lies opposite the third, fourth, fifth and sixth cervical vertebrae. The epiglottis is a flattened leaf-like sheet of elastic fibro cartilage, overhanging the entrance to the larynx. The larynx has four functions: (1) Respiratory (2) Sphincteric, (3) Protective reflexes and (4) Phonation.

Lung

The right and left lung are invaginated into the corresponding pleural cavities and are free, except at the root, where they are attached to the mediastinum. The general shape of the lung with its covering layer of visceral pleura is the same as that of the sac of parietal pleura in which it lies. The left lung is slightly smaller than the right lung due to the projection of the heart to the left. Although the right lung is larger than the left one, its vertical extent is less, since the right dome of the diaphragm lies at a higher level than that of the left dome owing to the greater mass of the liver on the right side. Lung tissue is soft, elastic and spongy. It contains numerous air sacs, which give it a characteristic feel and crackling sound when the lung is compressed between the finger and thumb. After birth, when respiration commences, the air-containing lungs floats in water, but before birth, the lung is solid and sinks in water. The highly vascular lung in early life has bright pink colour, but with advancing years, it may become grey or even black, especially in a town, through the progressive deposition of atmospheric dust and smoke in its substance.

The root of the lung contains the bronchi, the pulmonary and bronchial blood vessels, nerves, lymphatic vessels and nodes enclosed in the pleura. The bronchi are placed posterior and on each side, the bronchus has essentially the same relationship with the pulmonary artery.

PHYSIOLOGY OF THE RESPIRATORY SYSTEM

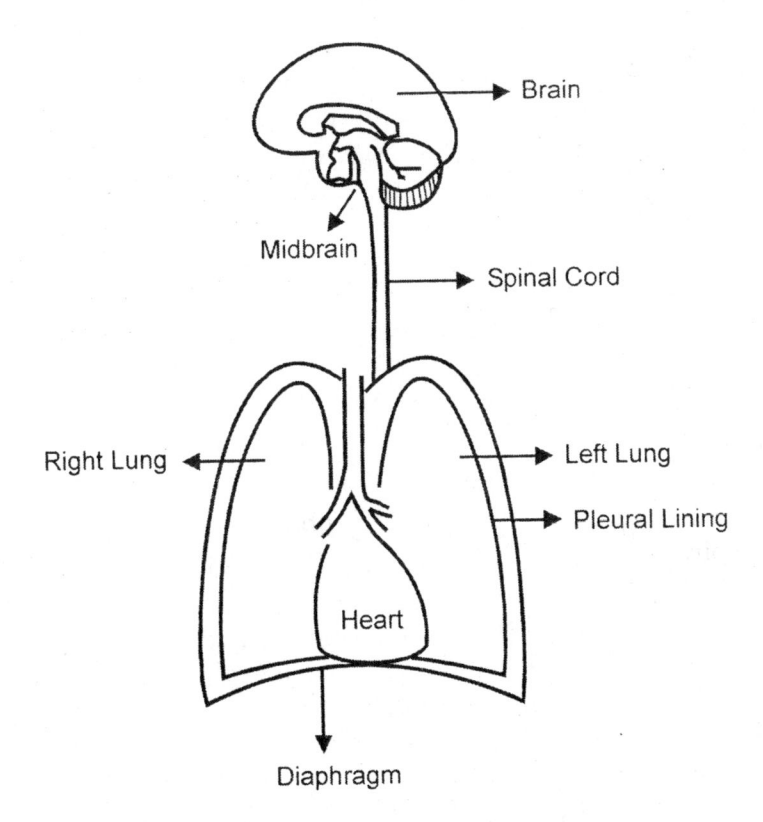

Humans need a continuous supply of oxygen for cellular respiration, and elimination of excess carbon dioxide, the poisonous waste product of this process. Gas exchange supports this cellular respiration by constantly supplying oxygen and removing carbon dioxide. The oxygen we need is derived from the Earth's atmosphere, which is 21% oxygen. This oxygen in the air is exchanged in the body by the respiratory surface. The alveoli in the lungs serve as the surface for gas exchange.

Although gas exchange takes place in the lungs, the respiratory system also includes two other components: the part of the central nervous system that controls our breathing, and the chest below.

The part of the nervous system that controls breathing is located in the mid-brain, also known as the brain stem. It is an area more primitive than the area of the brain responsible for thinking and motor movements, known as the brain cortex. Brain stem control of breathing is automatic and functions whether we think about it or not. However, drugs or some diseases may alter it. A relatively common cause of respiratory depression is an overdose with narcotics or sedatives.

Gas exchange in humans can be divided into five steps:

1. Breathing
2. External Respiration
3. Gas Transport
4. Internal Respiration
5. Cellular Respiration

Breathing consists of two phases, inspiration and expiration. During inspiration, the diaphragm and the intercostals muscles contract. The diaphragm moves downwards increasing the volume of the thoracic (chest) cavity, and the intercostals muscles pull the ribs up which results in expansion of the rib cage and further increasing this volume. This increase of volume lowers the air pressure in the alveoli to below atmospheric pressure. Because air always flows from a region of high pressure to a region of lower pressure, it rushes in through the respiratory tract and into the alveoli. This is called negative pressure breathing, changing the pressure inside the lungs relative to the pressure of the outside atmosphere. In contrast to inspiration, during expiration the' diaphragm and intercostal muscles relax. This returns the thoracic cavity to its original volume, increasing the air pressure in the lungs and forcing the air out. This process is facilitated by opening and closing of the muscles surrounding the bronchi and bronchioles, which is controlled by two groups of nerves called sympathetic and parasympathetic nerves. The sympathetic nerves help in the opening of the bronchi and bronchioles; the parasympathetic nerves cause their contraction.

The Respiratory Tree

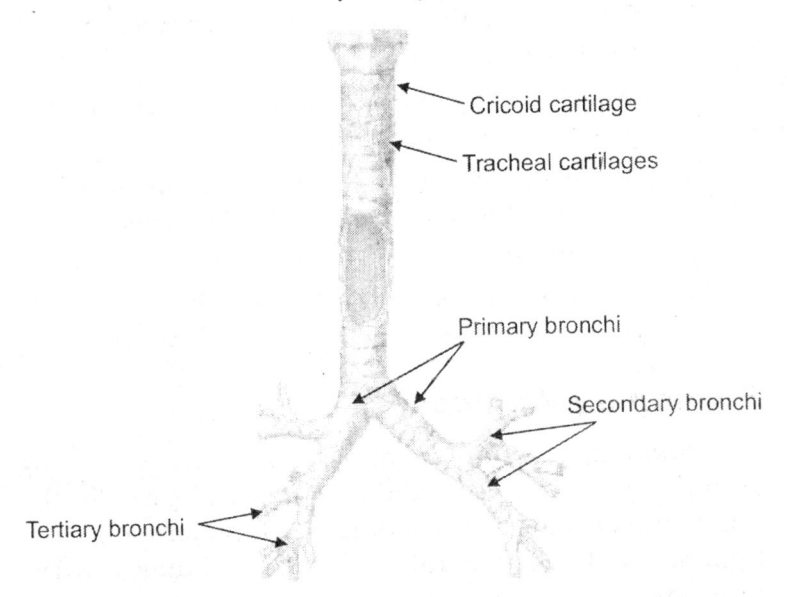

- Cricoid cartilage
- Tracheal cartilages
- Primary bronchi
- Secondary bronchi
- Tertiary bronchi

Thus the respiratory system is not only the lungs but also the central nervous system, chest wall (diaphragm, abdominal and intercostal muscles), and pulmonary circulation. The prime function of the system is to exchange gases between inspired air and venous blood, which is fulfilled with the sound and co-ordinated work of these prime or accessory organs or systems.

Respiratory in Humans — Some Principles

- In humans both diffusion and bulk flow move O_2 molecules between the external environment and actively metabolising tissues.
- This movement occurs in four (4) stages:
- Movement by bulk flow of the O_2 containing air to a thin, moist epithelium close to small blood vessels in the lungs.
    1. Diffusion of the O_2 across the epithelium into the blood.
    2. Movement by bulk flow with the circulating blood to the tissues where it will be used.
    3. Diffusion of the O_2 from the blood into the interstitial fluids, from which it diffuses into the individual cells.
    4. CO_2 — produced in the tissue cells, follows the reverse path as it is eliminated from the body.

Pulmonary Volumes

Pulmonary volumes are studied by recording graphically the changes of the volumes of gases in the lungs under different conditions of respiration in a Spirometer. It demonstrates the cyclic changes in the lung volume under each inspiratory and expiratory effort.

Introduction 17

A. SPIROMETER

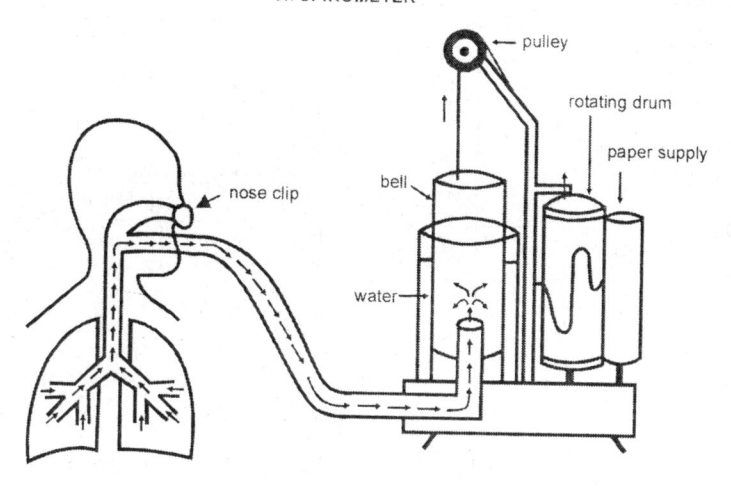

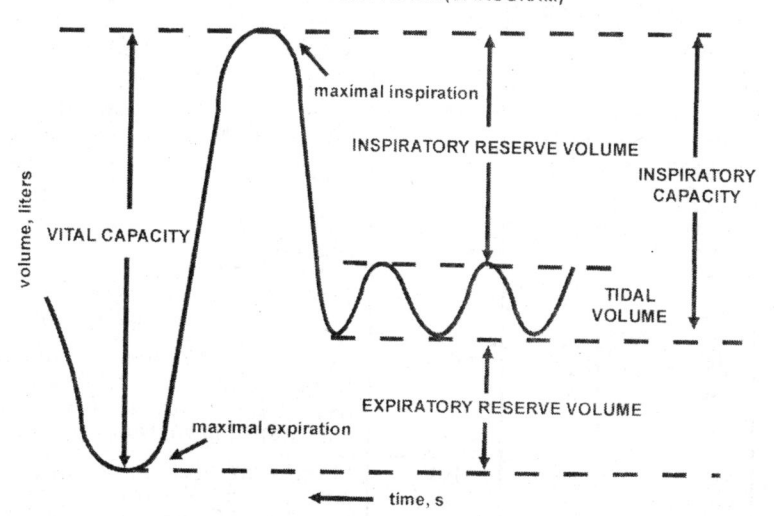

B. SPIROMETER TRACE (SPIROGRAM)

Following table shows the terms used in spirometric measurements.

Terms	Symbols	Descriptions
Vital capacity	VC	Maximal volume of air exhaled after forced inspiration (includes TV, IRV and ERV) 4800 ml in males 3100 ml in females
Tidal volume	TV	Volume of air inhaled or exhaled during quiet breathing. Appox. 500 ml
Inspiratory reserve volume	IRV	Maximal air that can be inhaled after a quiet inspiration. 2000 – 3300 ml
Expiratory reserve volume	ERV	Maximal air that can be breathed out after a quiet expiration. 1000 ml – 1500 ml
Residual volume	RV	Volume of air remaining in lungs after full expiration.
Inspiratory vital capacity	IVC	Maximal volume of air inhaled after full expiration. Appox. 3000 ml.
Forced expiratory volume, per time interval in seconds	FEV	Volume of air exhaled in a given period during a complete forced expiration (FVC).
Maximal expiratory	MEFR	Volume of air exhaled per second flow rate measured between the 200 ml and 1,200 ml volumes of the forced expiratory spirogram.
Maximal mid-expiratory flow	MMF	Volume of air per second exhaled during middle half of expired volume of forced expiratory spirogram.
Maximal voluntary ventilation	MVV	Maximum breathing capacity litre/minute. Subject can breathe with maximal voluntary effort (actual measurement for twelve seconds).

Introduction 19

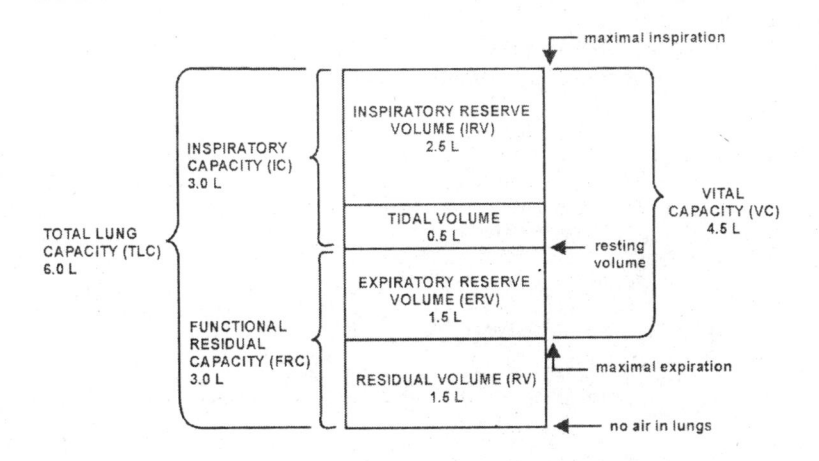

```
                              ┌── maximal inspiration
                  INSPIRATORY RESERVE
                     VOLUME (IRV)
      INSPIRATORY      2.5 L
      CAPACITY (IC)
      3.0 L                                VITAL
                                           CAPACITY (VC)
TOTAL LUNG          TIDAL VOLUME            4.5 L
CAPACITY (TLC)         0.5 L     ◄── resting
6.0 L                             volume
                  EXPIRATORY RESERVE
                     VOLUME (ERV)
      FUNCTIONAL       1.5 L
      RESIDUAL
      CAPACITY (FRC)
      3.0 L        RESIDUAL VOLUME (RV)  ── maximal expiration
                        1.5 L
                                     ── no air in lungs
```

The exchange of gases occurs between the membranes of the alveoli and the surrounding capillaries. The red blood cells are the vehicles that carry the carbon dioxide to and oxygen away from the alveoli.

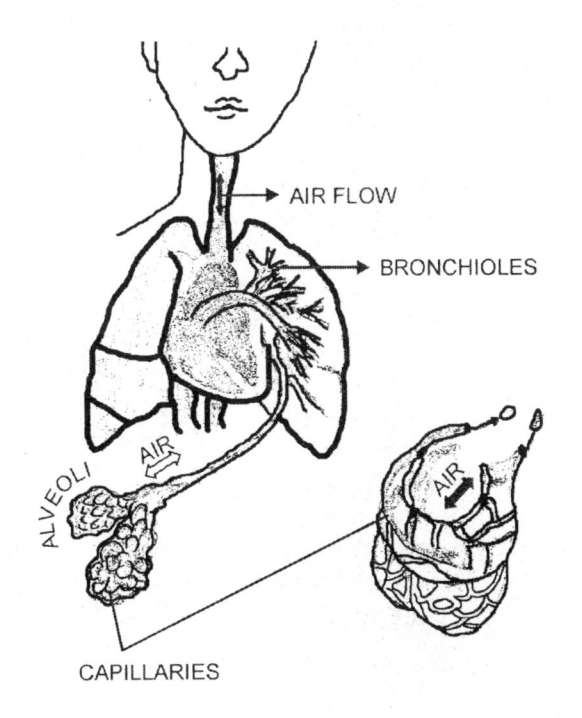

ALVEOLAR SAC STRUCTURE

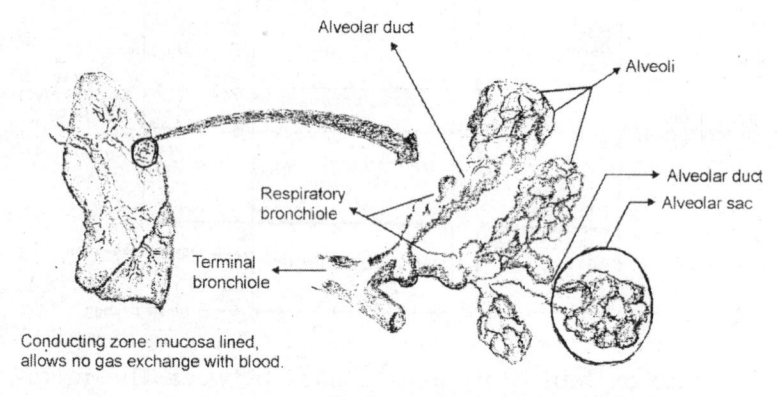

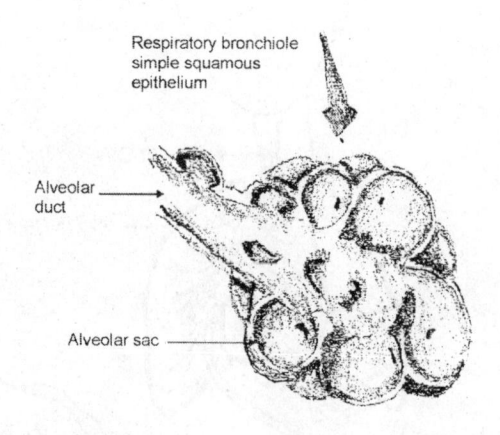

- Alveolar duct
- Alveoli
- Respiratory bronchiole
- Alveolar duct
- Alveolar sac
- Terminal bronchiole

Conducting zone: mucosa lined, allows no gas exchange with blood.

Respiratory zone: thin walled simple squamous epithelium, allows gas exchange with blood.

Respiratory bronchiole simple squamous epithelium

Alveolar duct

Alveolar sac

Alveoli are chambers of simple squamous epithelium. They connect to one another and to the alveolar duct. They form a sponge-like arrangement of gas filled spaces in lungs tissue.

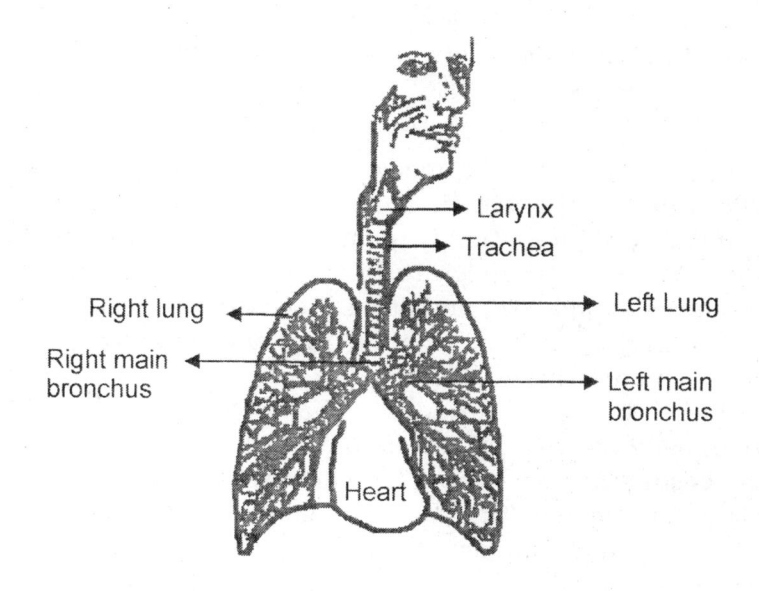

Arterial Blood Gases (ABG)

Blood gases measure the pH (acidity), oxygen content, and carbon dioxide content of the blood. Usually, blood gases are used to analyze the arterial blood. In rare cases, venous blood may be used. Also to determine the Acid/Base status of the blood. The results reported and predicted normally are:

- pH...................... 7.34 - 7.45
- PO_2...................... 80 - 100 mmHg
- PCO_2.................... 35 - 45 mmHg
- HCO_3.................... 22 - 26 mEq/L
- BE.......................... (-2) - (+2) mEq/L
- O_2 saturation.......... > 95%
- O_2 content.............. > 16 vol%
- $AaDO_2$................... 10 - 15 mmHg

Before we look at how these values change during an asthmatic attack, lets look at what bodily processes effect them.

pH is the negative log of the Hydrogen ion concentration. It's the measurement of the acidity or alkalinity of the blood. Most people know that the stomach produces acid, but many other processes do also. Muscles produces lactic acid, CO_2 in the blood produces a mild acid, and other processes produce acid. The kidneys control the production and elimination of Bicarbonate (where we get HCO_3), which the body uses to buffer the acids produced. The body maintains the acid/base balance by the kidneys retaining HCO_3 and increasing the rate of breathing (lowering CO_2) when the pH is low (acidic). The kidneys eliminate HCO_3 and the rate of breathing is lowered (too some extent) when the pH is high (alkaline).

PO_2 is the amount of Oxygen dissolved in the blood plasma, not the amount held in the red blood cells bound to haemoglobin. The PO_2 is affected by the amount of oxygen in the air we breathe (20.9% at sea level), our depth and rate of breathing, the amount of air reaching the alveoli, and the amount able to move across the Alveolar/Capillary barrier (the tissue between the alveoli holding the air and the capillaries holding the blood). The body has receptor that react to the levels of oxygen in the blood, these receptors tell the brain to increase or decrease respirations.

PCO_2 is the amount of Carbon Dioxide dissolved in the blood. The PCO_2, like PO_2, is affected by the depth and rate of breathing, and the amount of CO_2 that moves across the Alveolar/Capillary barrier. Note that CO_2 moves across this barrier easier than O_2. The amount of CO_2 increases with increased demands on the muscles, including those involved with respiration. There is also receptor for CO_2 that tell the brain to increase and decrease respiratory rate and depth. Note that these receptor are stronger than those for oxygen. The amount of carbon dioxide in the blood is the main drive to breathe.

HCO_3 is the bicarbonate ion and main buffering system of the body. The kidneys control the amounts of bicarbonate ions in the blood by eliminating or retaining the ion. CO_2 levels do affect HCO_3 to some extent, for every 10 to 15 mmHg increase of PCO_2 above 40 mmHg, the HCO_3 increases 1 mEq/L. For every 5 mmHg decrease below the normal for PCO_2, the HCO_3 decreases 1 mEq/L.

B.E., or Base Excess, also relates to bicarbonate, plus the buffering effects of haemoglobin are taken into effect. Base Excess uses PCO_2, HCO_3, and the haematocrit (amount of red blood cells) to calculate the non-respiratory part of the acid/base balance.

The O_2 Saturation is the total amount of oxygen bound to hemoglobin in the red blood cells in comparison to the total amount possible. For instance, if your O_2 Saturation is 50%, your hemoglobin is carrying only half of what it is capable of carrying.

The O_2 Content is the sum of the oxygen carried by the red blood cells (O_2 Sat) plus the amount dissolved in the plasma (PO_2). 99% of the oxygen carrying capacity of blood is the hemoglobin and 1% is dissolved in blood plasma. Therefore, O_2 Content is affected mostly by the amount of haemoglobin or red blood cells present in the blood stream. An anaemic person has a much lower capacity to carry oxygen than a normal person.

The $AaDO_2$, the Alveolar/Arterial Oxygen Difference is the difference of the amount of oxygen in the alveoli and arteries. Normally this difference is about 10 to 15 mmHg. If for some reason oxygen cannot make it across the alveolar/capillary barrier, this value and the difference between the oxygen in the lungs and the amount in the arteries increase.

What do the test results mean?

There are several values that are measured in an ABG. Each of the values has a set range that is considered normal. If any of the main values becomes severely abnormal, it may result in death.

The **pH** is one of the main parts of this test. This is a measure of the level of acid in the blood. Acid levels may be too high with:

- kidney failure or damage
- certain cases of uncontrolled diabetes
- exposure to certain toxic substances, such as a drug overdose
- shock, which may occur from heart failure, serious infections, or massive blood or fluid loss
- breathing troubles, such as lung infections, asthma, emphysema, or not breathing fast enough
- certain medications

Acid levels may be too low from:
- dehydration
- certain types of kidney problems
- breathing too fast, such as when a person has a panic disorder
- excessive vomiting
- salt imbalances, which may be from a hormone problem in the body
- certain medications

If the pH is abnormal, the other parts of the test can help determine the reason. For example, if the acid level in the body is too high, it could be from breathing or metabolism problems. It is important to know what is the cause of the high acid level, as the treatment is often different. If the acid level is too high because of a breathing problem, the person may need extra oxygen or even a ventilator. If the acid level is too high from metabolism problems, a person may need to be hooked up to a blood-filtering machine, or may need antibiotics or other drugs.

The breathing parts of the test are the oxygen and carbon dioxide levels in the blood. The job of the lungs is to take in oxygen and get rid of carbon dioxide. If some type of breathing or respiratory problem is present, these values will be abnormal. The oxygen level can also be used to check if a person is getting enough oxygen or whether they need extra oxygen.

The part of the test that measures the bicarbonate level in the blood will determine whether there is a metabolism problem. If a metabolism problem is present, this value will be abnormal.

There are other minor parts of the test that may be monitored by a healthcare provider in certain situations.

The healthcare provider must look at the pH, breathing, and metabolic parts of the test together. This allows the provider to sort out different problems in a person's body.

There are **four main** states expressed by ABGs other than normal, they are Respiratory Acidosis, Respiratory Alkalosis, Metabolic Acidosis, and Metabolic Alkalosis.

Respiratory Acidosis - is basically too much CO_2 in the blood and causes the pH to drop (become more acidic). This is a sign of respiratory distress and/or disease. If this condition worsens and is not dealt with it will lead to respiratory failure. Given time the HCO_3 and B.E. will increase to compensate for the increased CO_2. This is called Compensated Respiratory Acidosis.

Respiratory Alkalosis - is too little CO_2 in the blood, this causes the pH to rise (become more alkaline). Some of the causes can be hypoxemia (low PO_2 and O_2 Saturation), pain, emotional distress, injuries to the brain, etc. If the person is hypoxic, correcting the underlying cause, in bronchospasm, inflammation of the airways, and thick mucus, will allow more oxygen to make it to the blood stream. The person's breathing will return to normal and CO_2 levels will also return to normal. If left uncorrected and does not get worse, the HCO_3 and B.E. will over time correct the pH, you then have a compensated Respiratory Alkalosis.

Metabolic Acidosis and Metabolic Alkalosis are related to processes that cause HCO_3 and B.E. to rise and fall, thus causing the pH to rise or fall.

Some of the possible causes of Metabolic Acidosis (low HCO_3, B.E.)- are Diarrhoea, Renal disease, Ketoacidosis, Lactic acidosis (lack of oxygen in the tissues), and poisoning. The respiratory system will try to compensate for this condition by increasing respiratory rate to blow off more CO_2. If successful, the pH will return to normal and you have a Compensated Metabolic Acidosis. As respiratory muscles tire, this condition can decompensate.

Metabolic Alkalosis (excess HCO_3, B.E.) - can be caused by Hypokalemia (too little potassium in the blood), Hypochloremia (too little chloride), persistent vomiting, Diuretic therapy, and Steroid therapy. Metabolic Alkalosis tends to remain uncompensated in the awake person, since the demand to breathe does not lessen to any great degree.

A person can have a mixture of any of these acid/base disorders.

Initially we may not even notice the changes taking place, a little cough or a slight wheeze. But in the lungs these changes are affecting our entire body. As the airways narrow in response to **Asthma Triggers**, the amount of Oxygen getting down to the alveoli is starting to drop. The body compensates by increasing the respiratory rate. As the attack worsens to the point where we start considering taking our "Rescue Medication", usually a Beta 2-Agonist like Ventrolin, our breathing rate is high enough to drop our CO_2 levels and move the pH up to cause a slight Respiratory Alkalosis. In most cases the bronchodilator works and everything returns to normal. Our blood gases will have a pH slightly above 7.45, a PCO_2 slightly below 35 mmHg, a PO_2 in the 80s, and everything else pretty much normal.

Many times the usual medications don't work out. The attack worsens, coughing increases and so does shortness of breath. Some alveoli are cut off from receiving air, and the blood goes by them unoxygenated, putting more dependance on the ones still open. The lungs work harder to keep up with the demand for oxygen, the muscles of the respiratory system work harder and in the process produce more CO_2. But at this point we have the reserves to handle the extra work and CO_2. Our blood gases now have a pH 7.50 or above, our PCO_2 is in the 20s, our PO_2 may now be well into the 60s, and the HCO_3 and B.E. just now starting to compensate slightly. This should be attention-seeking situation. If proper treatment is administered at this point many problems can be averted, procrastination or lack of the needed medical care can lead to grave consequences.

In couple of hours now since the attack started our blood gases are starting to do a "U" turn. We've reached the limit of our reserves, but the demands are still mounting. Many areas of our lungs may be shut off from air reaching them; more and more blood passes through the lungs unoxygenated.

Our respiratory muscle are beginning to tire, so we breathe less rapidly and our PCO_2 starts to rise back into the normal range, our PO_2 looks better because of the nasal cannula, and our pH is coming back to normal with rising PCO_2. The HCO_3 and B.E. are still a little low.

At this point if the attack is not brought under control the downward spiral will accelerate and things begin to happen very quickly. As the PCO_2 continues to climb above the normal range we will become lethargic, possibly losing consciousness, diaphoretic (profuse sweating), possibly cyanotic (bluish coloring) around the lips and nail beds, our PO_2 will start to plummet and with it our pH. Our respiratory muscles are exhausted, our airways are so swollen that very little air can pass, and respiratory failure is right around the corner. Respiratory failure is the complete collapse of the respiratory system, in which one stops breathing. If we are lucky we wake up on a ventilator, if not, we may not wake up at all.

If asthma attacks are dealt promptly and appropriately many deaths can be averted.

2

MAIN DISEASES OF THE RESPIRATORY SYSTEM

HYPERVENTILATION SYNDROME

HVS is a condition in which minute ventilation exceeds metabolic demands, resulting in hemodynamic and chemical changes that produce characteristic symptoms.

Symptoms of HVS and panic disorder overlap considerably, although both the conditions remain distinct. Approximately 50% of patients with panic disorder and 60% of patients with agoraphobia manifest hyper-ventilation as part of their symptomatology, whereas only 25% of patients with HVS manifest panic disorder.

Pathophysiology

HVS occurs in acute and chronic forms.

Acute HVS accounts for only 1% of cases but is diagnosed more easily.

Chronic HVS can present with respiratory, cardiac, neurological, or GI symptoms without any clinically apparent over breathing.

The underlying mechanism by which some patients develop hyperventilation is unknown, but theories abound. Certain stressors have been identified which provoke an exaggerated respiratory response including emotional distress, sodium lactate, caffeine, isoproterenol, cholecystokinin, and CO_2.

Part of the explanation for HVS lies in the mechanics of breathing. Normal tidal volumes range from 35-45% of vital capacity at rest. The elastic recoil of the chest wall resists hyperinflation of the lungs beyond that level, and inspiratory volumes beyond this level are considered as effort or dyspnoea.

Patients with HVS tend to breathe by using the upper thorax rather than the diaphragm, resulting in chronically overinflated lungs. When stress induces a need to take a deep breath, the deep breathing is perceived as dyspnoea. The sensation of dyspnoea creates anxiety, which encourages more deep breathing, and a vicious cycle is created.

Patients with panic disorder have a lower threshold for the fight or flight response and tend to manifest with primarily psychiatric complaints, such as fear of death, impending doom, or claustrophobia. Patients with HVS tend to focus on somatic complaints related to the physiologic changes produced by hyperventilation. The initiating stimulus and the abnormal stress response may be identical in each group but are expressed differently.

Mortality / Morbidity

- Death is extremely rare. A leftward shift in the HbO_2 dissociation curve and vasospasm related to low PCO_2 might cause myocardial ischaemia in patients with coronary artery disease and HVS.
- Certain patients are affected psychologically by their symptoms, and many patients carry false diagnoses. The real danger for patients with HVS is that they suffer complications from unneeded investigations (eg. angiography) or treatment (eg. thrombolytics). Withholding such therapy may be extremely difficult in a patient with crushing chest pain, dyspnoea, and/or suggestive electrocardiogram (ECG) changes.

- One study reported a series of 45 patients with chest pain who had normal coronary arteries on angiography. These patients ultimately were diagnosed as having HVS. Over a 3.5-year average follow-up period, 67% of the patients had made subsequent ED visits for chest pain, and 40% of the patients had been readmitted to rule out myocardial infarction.
- Clearly HVS not only produces severe and genuine discomfort for the patient, it also accounts for considerable medical expenses in excluding more serious pathology.

Dr. Mehta suggests that in this condition one should inhale the same air as he is expelling by making a sort of cup by putting two hands together near the nose. This will allow the same air to be inhaled again. According to his experience this helps a lot — may be due to the CO_2 re intake to some extent and also the body doesn't have to re adjust the temperature of inhaled air, as it is equivalent to body temperature.

Rhinitis (common cold), influenza, tonsillitis, bronchitis, bronchiectasis, pneumonia and tuberculosis are some of the common diseases of the respiratory system. Before going into the detailed description of asthma, it is necessary to provide general information regarding these diseases, as they are related to the subject.

RHINITIS (PINASA)

Heaviness of the head, anorexia, thin (watery) nasal discharge, feeble voice and fequent spitting are the features of the early stage of Pinasa.

In the later stages the discharge becomes thick, has the features of amakapha (mucopurulent) and keep the nasal passage blocked and the voice and the appearnace of the patient becomes normal.

It is an inflammatory condition of the mucous membrane of nose characterized by sneezing, watery discharge from the nose, and obstruction of the nasal passages. It may be associated with conjunctional and pharyngeal itching, lacrimation and sinusitis.

It is commonly caused by exposure to pollens, contact with household dust and animal wastes, sudden climatic changes, cold, fumes and bacterial infections.

General symptoms of rhinitis also may include mild to moderate fever, severe headache, malaise etc.

Altogether this is an irritating condition which is not dangerous, hence common cold is generally taken lightly by both the patients and the physicians which is evident from the well-known adage: "If you take medicine for a cold, it gets cured in a week; otherwise it takes seven days". But, if this benign condition is neglected for a long time, it can lead to more serious, allergic conditions like allergic bronchitis, asthma etc.

INFLUENZA (PRATISHYAYA)

In chapter 26 of charak chikitsasthan the causative factors of pratishyaya are described which includes suppression of natural urges, inhalatin of dust, abnormal seasonal changes, excessive sleep, exposure to dew, vapours or smoke.

Vata aggravated by these factors in the head, the site of viscid dosa (i.e. Kapha) gives rise to pratishyay.

According to Sushruta Vata and other dosas (i.e. Pitta and Kapha) singly or all together as also Rakta, vitiated by their respective exciting factors accumulate in the head to give rise to various symptoms of influenza.

It is an acute viral, infectious disease, characterised by a sudden onset headache, fever, chills, muscular pains, cough, and sore throat. Prominent features of influenza are irritation and inflammation of the mucosa of the nose, pharynx and larynx, bleeding from the nose and a dry hacking cough. In uncomplicated influenza the acute illness generally resolves in 2-5 days and most patients recover within 1 week. The most common complication of influenza is pneumonia, which is of various types. Patients with chronic lung disease or cardiac disease and elderly individual are at a particular risk for secondary bacterial pneumonia.

Influenza generally strikes at the junction of change of seasons with an incubation period of 3-10 days. People who are prone to influenza are those who suffer from constipation.

TONSILLITIS
(KANTHASHALUK AND TUNDIKERI)

Kanthashaluka according to Sushruta is rough nodular swelling in the throat that occurs due to Kapha. Tundikeri is an acute swelling due to Kapha and Rakta and is associated with pricking pain and burning sensation and with a tendency for suppuration.

It is an inflammatory condition of the tonsils – small rounded mass of mainly lymphoid tissues behind the tongue on either side of the pharynx, acting as barriers to infection. The organism Streptococcus haemolyticus mainly causes it. The onset of tonsillitis is characterized by pain in the throat while swallowing, sensation of chill and fever. In severe cases of tonsillitis, there may also be difficulty in breathing. On physical examination, the tonsils are enlarged and sometimes may have a thin curd like layer on it, which indicates severity of infection. This condition should not be ignored specifically in children below the age of 18 for this may be a sign of rheumatic fever.

BRONCHITIS
(SHWASNALIKA SHOTHA)

This is a type of Kaphaj Kasa (cough) which starts with irritation in respiratory tract followed by inflammation of bronchioles and exudation. Its features as described in Sushrut S.52 are stickiness in the oral cavity, excess of Kapha in the body, a feeling of heaviness and itching sesnation with severe bouts of cough producing a thick expectoration.

It is an inflammatory condition of the mucous membranes of the trachea and bronchi, caused by viruses, bacteria and external irritants as in the case of allergic bronchitis. It can be chronic bronchitis, simple or of the muco purulent type. It can be chronic asthmatic bronchitis too. The latter is characterised by cough and increased mucus secretion associated with dyspnoea and wheezing with acute respiratory infections or exposure to inhaled irritants. In its acute form it may give rise to high temperature, breathlessness and loss of appetite. The chronic forms of bronchitis if not treated in time may lead to chronic obstructive air-way diseases, (COAD), with chronic expiratory airflow obstruction. COAD is a progressive disorders even when contributing factors are eliminated and aggressive therapy is instituted.

BRONCHIECTASIS
(SHWASANALIKA PRASARA)

It is a condition characterised by chronic permanent dilatation of one or more bronchi, which impairs the drainage of bronchial secretions and leads to persistent infection in the affected segment or lobe.

PNEUMONIA (SHWASNAK JWARA)

This falls in the category of continous or Remittent type of Viasham Jwar. It is the Kapha dominant Intermittent fever in which the rise of temprature is continuous without any break for a period of seven, ten or tweleve days along with other symptoms like difficulty in breathig with abnormal sounds, cough, painful respiration etc.

Some authorities hold the view that Shwasnak Jwar is due to infection (affliction) by organisms (Superhuman agencies / evil spirits).

It is an infection of the pulmonary parenchyma caused by various bacterial species, viruses, fungi and parasites. Compromised hosts are particularly vulnerable to pulmonary infections caused by a variety of pathogens. The characteristic finding includes fever and cough with or without sputum. On chest examination, there is dullness on percussion. Decreased breath sounds, bronchial breath sounds or rales are found on auscultation. Associated finding can include pleuritic chest pain, rigors, dyspnoea, muscular pains, headache and diarrhoea.

TUBERCULOSIS (RAJYAKSHMA)

Obstruction of nutrition carrying channels predominantly by the Kapha dosa and also excessive loss of semen leads to depletion of all the tissues (Dhatus) of the body and the patient develops features like dyspnoea, bodyache, spiting of mucus, corryza, dyspepsia, haemoptysis and generalised rise of body temprature.

Tuberculosis is a disease caused by an organism "*mycobacterium tuberculi.*" Slight rise in temperature or low-grade fever generally in the evenings, night sweats, cough with blood tinged sputum, haemoptysis, loss of appetites, and fatigue is the main clinical presentations of tuberculosis. It is one of the most contagious diseases to affect mankind. Worldwide, there are more than 30 million cases of active tuberculosis and there are 10 million new cases annually. It is estimated that 3 million people die of tuberculosis each year. Main factors responsible for the occurrence of the disease are malnutrition, unhygienic conditions at home or/and work, low resistance due to various factors like poor ventilation, chronic diseases, metabolic disorders like diabetes, AIDS etc. In the early stage, the disease primarily involves the lungs and gives rise to the above said symptoms. But if proper intervention on time is not made, it may lead to affection of other organs i.e. extra pulmonary tuberculosis like pleural effusion, pericarditis, peritonitis, endobronchial tuberculosis, meningeal tuberculosis etc. In the terminal stage of pulmonary tuberculosis, there is a formation of cavity in lungs leading to extensive haemorrhage and death.

3

ASTHMA

Asthma is a very common disorder with an estimated four to five percent of the population being affected. It is perhaps the only common treatable condition that is increasing in terms of prevalence, severity and mortality, especially in children.

Asthma is a chronic inflammatory condition of the airways. In susceptible individuals this inflammation causes recurrent episodes of coughing, wheezing, chest tightness, and difficult breathing. Inflammation makes the airways sensitive to stimuli such as, chemical irritant, tobacco smoke, cold air, or exercise. When exposed to these stimuli, the airways may become swollen, constricted, filled with mucus, and hypersensitive to stimuli.

The inflammation causes associated increase in existing airway hyper responsiveness to variety of cold air and virus. Exposure of patients to these stimuli provokes a variety of changes in airways including broncho constriction, airway oedema, chronic mucus plug formation and airway remodelling. The recurrent episodes of wheezing, breathlessness, chest tightness and coughing experienced by patient with asthma, particularly at night and in early morning, is usually associated with airflow obstruction.

Asthma attacks all age groups but often starts in childhood. It is a disease characterized by recurrent attacks of breathlessness and wheezing, which vary in severity and frequency from person to person. In an individual, they may occur from hour to hour and day to day.

This condition is due to inflammation of the air passages in the lungs and affects the sensitivity of the nerve endings in the airways so they become easily irritated. In an attack, the lining of the passages swell causing the airways to narrow and reducing the flow of air in and out of the lungs.

Asthma, technically called bronchial asthma, is a disease of the bronchial tubes that lead from the windpipe, or trachea, into the lungs. The bronchial tubes ordinarily do not furnish any marked resistance to the entrance or exit of air. However, in asthmatic attacks, the bronchial tubes tend to close down, causing asthmatic wheezing. In severe attack, the sufferer seems almost to be suffocating. He apparently uses all his strength just trying to breathe. He becomes pale and bluish and often perspires. Fortunately, most attacks are mild and do not last long. Many of them can be prevented or stopped by medical treatment.

Bronchial asthma is a chronic illness marked by these attacks. In severe cases, the bronchial tubes become swollen and ofter greater resistance to treatment. Plugs of clinging mucus may form in the tubes and cause chronic irritation and coughing. They are dislodged and brought up as sputum. If the attacks are frequent, prolonged, and severe, the lung tissue is damaged. This puts a strain on the heart. The average case of asthma is mild and more of a recurrent nuisance than a threat to health. It is always essential to get and follow competent medical advice, especially in the cases of young persons, before asthma can damage the heart or lungs.

The resulting airflow limitation is reversible, either spontaneously or with treatment; when asthma therapy is adequate, inflammation can be reduced over the long term, symptoms can usually be controlled, and most asthma related problems prevented.

OCCURRENCE

Asthma can occur at any age but the frequency and degree of their symptoms may vary. Some people have only an occasional attack i.e. mild in degree and a brief duration and otherwise are entirely free of symptoms. Others have mild coughing and wheezing most of the time, triggered by several attacks following exposure to known allergens, infections or certain stress conditions.

Asthma can go unnoticed in people with the history of eczema and family history of other allergy disorders and who suffer from recurrent wheezing.

Asthma is not a public health problem in developed countries. In developing countries, however, the incidence of the disease varies greatly.

THE HUMAN AND ECONOMIC BURDEN

Mortality due to asthma is not comparable in size to the day-to-day effects of the disease. Asthma tends to occur in epidemics and affects mostly young people. The human and economic burden associated with this condition is severe. The cost of asthma to the society could be reduced to a large extent through concerted inter-national and national action.

EPIDEMIOLOGICAL EVIDENCE

Latest studies reveal that nearly 90% of childhood asthma have atopic features. Co-existent AR or chronic sinusitis may worsen asthma clinically. AR and asthma are closely linked. AR, sinusitis, ocular allergy and asthma can all co-exist or follow one another in succession. In general population in India, atopic disorders are common and seen in nearly 25%, most of which are naso-bronchial allergies. Chronic sinusitis clinically is associated strongly with asthma and naso-bronchial allergy. In earlier stages AR is often associated with ocular allergy.

40% of AR cases had associated asthma, while 50% to 80% cases of asthma had AR.

98.9% incidence of AR are such that where allergy is associated with asthma. Even in non-allergic asthma, AR is also high (78.4%). So it's concluded that a 'chronic allergic total airway disease syndrome' exists. The level of IgE in blood (a marker of allergy) rises both in AR and in asthma, whether extrinsic and intrinsic, as compared to normal controls.

CHILDHOOD-ONSET ASTHMA

This is closely linked with the presence of eczema, hay fever, urticaria and migraine in the patient or in close relatives. People with this kind of family history are called atopic. If both parents have a history of atopy then the chances of the child being affected is 50%; if one parent is affected, the chance is 30%; and if neither parent is affected, the chance is approximately 12%. Childhood asthma may very often be preceded for several months or even years by episodic coughing which later develops into wheezy bronchitis and then eventually into asthma. Such children often have a history of slow recovery from upper respiratory tract viral infections as well as a personal or family history of atopy.

ADULT-ONSET ASTHMA

Adult-onset asthma is more common in women than men. There are two broad types. In the first there are no obvious reasons for the asthmatic attacks. In the second, there are fairly obvious trigger factors that precipitate attacks. The sufferer should avoid such triggers but, even so, new allergens will continue to be detected, to be added to the list of external or environmental causes of the condition. Common triggers include:

- **Inhaled allergens** — Commonly inhaled allergens include the house-dust mite, animal danders, pollens, particularly grass, mould spores.
- **Irritant gases** — Including cigarette smoke.
- **Ingested allergens** — Foods; drugs, e.g. aspirin, colour medicines (pills, capsules and syrups); food additives; yeast and moulds on food.
- **Infecting organisms** — Either due to the infection itself or an allergy to the organism.
- **Temperature changes** — Especially cold humid air.
- **Changes in the weather.**
- **Exercise.**
- **Emotional stress.**
- **Hormonal changes.**
- **Certain chemicals in the work place.**

EMBRYOLOGY

"Shonitphena prabhvha phupphusha." (Su.sh)

We get a hint in Sushruta Samhita sharir sthan chapter 4 about the formation of lungs. To our surprise Acharya says that the lungs are formed by the froth of the blood. Being Ayurveda scientists it's our duty to expound the truth behind this philosophy as we know it's true.

In this case we have two things which are to be explored: Blood and Froth.

Sushruta says that blood (shonita) is a composition

of five elements like all substances. The qualities of shonita as per five elements are:

Earth	—	Fishy odour
Water	—	Liquidity
Fire	—	Redness
Air	—	Pulsation
Ether	—	Lightness.

Along with these properties Earth also provides compactness.

In Sharir sthana, Charaka says "Dwyo shleshmabhuvo" means these Lungs are the resultant of Shleshma (Kapha). Also we know that kapha is made up of Earth and Water.

So Earth and Water give the base for the formation of lungs. Then probably some movement due to air starts in the water (liquids) to produce some froth.

- Here Earth element - makes - surface tension (the tendency of molecules in a fluid to be pulled towards the centre of the fluid).
- The Water element with Air – makes - surfactants (the substances that reduce surface tension).

The free-floating bubbles are spherical because that's the smallest surface possible for a given amount of bubble.

Alveoli have the same shape as a bubble and behave much the same way. Physicists say that the colours of bubbles are related to the thickness of soap film.

There is a surfactant in our lungs so the Air we breathe can expand tiny little Air sacs way down inside.

These surfactants prevent water droplets from blocking airways. Body uses surfactants to reduce surface tension in the mucous lining of the pulmonary alveoli. These Alveoli contract and expand at an average of 15000 times per day in a normal adult.

WHO ARE PRONE TO ASTHMA?

Asthma is related to atopy. Atopy is a familial tendency to develop hypersensitivity after exposure to allergens.

Atopy is an autosomal dominant trait. Atopic individuals frequently suffer from allergic rhinitis, bronchial asthma, atopic dermatitis, eczema or urticaria. These disorders are type I immune disorders, mediated by immunoglobulin E (IgE). All atopics do not develop the disease. The cause of atopic individuals to develop the disease is not exactly known.

NATURE OF ASTHMA

Asthma is a frightening condition, which can seriously impede one's ability to breathe, and suddenly rob the individual of the most important nutrient of all – oxygen. Whereas asthma has not been a serious health problem in pre industrial societies, development of large industrial complexes has clearly increased prevalence of this condition. The socioeconomic status is another important factor affecting the prevalence of asthma.

In view of the fact that air pollution is conjectured to play a major role in the prevalence of asthma, and that asthma is believed to be a disease of civilization, much effort has been directed towards improving the quality of the air we breathe.

The process of breathing in and out is effortless, thus hardly noticeable, and therefore, often taken for granted. Through a life span, consider the new born's *first gasp for air* outside mother's womb, signifying the wonderful act of entry into this world, the infant's first *vocal sounds and lisps* that express emotions enabling communication with the world, and finally, the inevitable act of dying, or expiration, marked by giving the spirit away with the *last breath* - all tied to the respiratory tract.

This is true because respiratory difficulties constitute the commonest cause of morbidity in newborn babies. Pediatrician judges the condition by **APGAR** scoring system in which respiration is an important factor.

Table: Clinical respiratory distress scoring system.

Score	0	1	2
1. Respiration (rate/min)	None	Slow, irregular	Good, crying
2. Heart rate/min.	Absent	< 100	> 100
3. Colour of the body	Blue or pale	Body pink, extremities blue	pink
4. Muscle tone of the extremities	Flaccid	Some flexion	Actively moving
5. Reflex stimulation	No response	Grimace	Cries, coughs or sneezes.

Foetal lung development

Role of *Panchmahabhuta* (five elements) in Foetal lungs growth.

1. Aakash (ether) – the formation of cavities like alveoli etc.
2. Vayu (air) – continuous foetal breathing movements.
3. Teja (fire) – colour of the lungs and temperature maintenance.
4. Jala (water) – the amniotic fluid.
5. Prithvi (earth) – the solidity and shape to the trachea, bronchioles and lungs in total.

Arterial blood gases (vayu associated with agni) reflects

i. Pulmonary

ii. Cardiac

iii. Metabolic status of the new born

Oxygen (*prana-vayu*) is carried in the blood (part of *agni*) in chemical combination with haemoglobin (*part of agni*) and in solution form (*part of jala*). Most of the oxygen is bound with haemoglobin and blood.

Foetal lung growth is dependent upon foetal breathing movements and quantity of the amniotic fluid.

The clinical diagnosis of respiratory distress in the newborn is suspected when the respiratory rate is more than 60 per minute in a quiet resting baby and there are inspiratory costal recessions or expiratory grunt.

The physiological function (of gas exchange) of respiratory system are not carried out until after birth. The respiratory tract, diaphragm and lungs do form early in embryonic development. In the head/neck region, the pharynx forms a major arched cavity within the pharyngeal arches. The lungs go through 4 distinct phases of development and late in foetal development respiratory motions and amniotic fluid are thought to have a role in lung maturation.

Blood supply

- Pulmonary system is not "functional" until after birth
- 6th aortic arch arteries generate pulmonary arteries
- Veins drain into pulmonary vein then left atrium
- Branches from dorsal aorta generate bronchial arteries

Lung histology

- Month 3rd to 6th — lungs appear glandular
- End of month 6th — alveolar cells type 2 appear and begin to secrete surfactant
- Month 7th — respiratory bronchioles proliferate and end in alveolar ducts and sacs

    The epithelial components of the lungs develop

from an out pouching of the laryngotracheal tube that projects inferiorly and then laterally into the pericardio-peritoneal sac which later on forms the pleura. The main lung buds on each side ramify into successively smaller elements of the bronchial tree. The surrounding mesoderm migrates into this tissue to form cartilage and muscle.

The capillary bed develops at 23-24 weeks; this defines the limit of viability of birth. The definitive alveoli don't appear until term and then continue to develop until age 8-11 years. The majority of an adult's alveoli are produced in this time. Surfactant begins to be produced from six months in utero.

Lung fluid is being produced at a rate of 300 ml/day at term; this fills the lungs to their resting volume of 100 mls. Also, it is contributed to by the swallowing of amniotic fluid; this may be forcibly exhaled at birth or absorbed into the lungs.

The combination of breathing movements and sufficient liquor volume aids proper development of lungs.

Conditions such as oligohydramnios leads to pulmonary hypoplasia, for example, in Potter's syndrome.

Amniotic fluid thus have a major role in lung maturation.

Both the physical and mental characteristic of the child depends upon the state of mother during the period of gestation.

According to *Vagbhatta* the resort to action and use of articles of food by the mother which tend to excite vata may contribute to malformations and deformities.

Diet during pregnancy

3rd month – diet consisting of sweet, cold, liquids.

Particularly she should be fed on boiled shashtika rice with milk.

4th,5th 6th month- Shastika rice with curd, milk and ghee respectively.

Properties of Amniotic fluid are more or less similar to that of milk, ghee or any other milk products and shastika rice. Sufficient liquor amni aids in proper lung development as normal volume of amniotic fluid (AF) provides the foetus with some more important benefits:

- Cushioning effect that protects the foetus from direct trauma and the umbilical cord from compression that could impede normal fetoplacental circulation.
- It contains bacteriostatic properties which can protect the intrauterine environment from infection.
- It can serve as a short term fluid and nutrient supply.
- It is needed for proper development of gastrointestinal, musculoskeletal and pulmonary systems.

As by this we understand that proper intake of fluids is necessary for the replenishing of Amniotic fluid; here we can compensate this fluid intake with the intake of milk as it can serve other purposes also like providing Calcium etc.

Extra fluids are not only necessary to increase the blood volume by 40 percent and to keep refilling the pool of amniotic fluid; they are also necessary for the overall well being during pregnancy. Drinking lots of water and other fluids helps keep the skin soft and smooth. More fluids in the diet put more fluids in bowels, lessening constipation. Keeping the body primed with extra fluids helps move along and dilute the body's waste products and causes urination more frequently, lessening the risk of urinary tract infections. Eight 8-ounce glasses of fluid a day keeps the body and baby well hydrated. Avoid caffeine and alcohol, since these substances have a diuretic effect, robbing the body of fluids.

CHAIN REACTION LEADING TO ASTHMA

According to the definition utilized by many physicians, asthma is not a disease but rather a syndrome, which unlike a disease cannot be attributed to one specific cause, but rather to several causes. Most commonly, an asthma attack is described as an allergic reaction of the respiratory tract leading to a drastic narrowing of air passages, triggered by a variety of air pollutants commonly described as allergens. There are other causes leading to the frightening experience of asthma including abnormal response to aspirin and some other NSAID (non-steroidal anti-inflammatory drugs) i.e. aspirin induced asthma, and abnormal response to exercise, i.e. exercise induced asthma.

It is likely that asthma attacks triggered by different factors have different mechanisms that ultimately lead to the narrowing of air passages. Three leading theories are currently discussed to explain asthma mechanisms:

- The first one, and the most popular one, is that asthma is a fundamentally allergic sequence due to a wrongful response of the immune (defence) system to a challenge, e.g. by inhaled pollutants.
- The second theory is the "neurogenic hypothesis" that asthma attacks are precipitated by a sudden spasm of smooth muscles in the air passages due to imbalance within the nervous system, i.e. autonomous nervous system which regulates smooth muscles via ß-receptors etc.
- The third theory nicknamed "myogenic hypothesis" explains that white cells migrating to walls of air passages make the smooth muscles hyperactive and prone to sudden spasms leading to an asthma attack.

EFFECT OF ALLERGENS ON ASTHMA

The process of respiration involves inhalation and exhalation of air into and from the lungs and is affected through a complex mechanism coordinated by the respiratory center of the brain. The ribs, muscles attached to the rib cage, and a muscular membrane-like structure, known as diaphragm, separating the abdomen from the thorax facilitate the process of respiration, during the inhalation or exhalation of air. In addition to this mechanism, the walls of the bronchial tree are equipped with bronchial muscles that either dilate or contract the air passages. In fact, there is a circadian rhythm operating the bronchial muscles which results in maximal dilation of air passages at about 6 p.m. and maximal constriction of air passages at 6 a.m. This explains why asthma attacks are more severe in the morning hours than in the evening. The other recognized factors that affect bronchial muscles and respiration are emotional and physical factors, such as altitude, temperature, and humidity of air, mostly by influencing the receptors dispersed in the walls of air passages. It is known, for example, that drugs stimulating ß-receptors cause dilation of air passages, while ß-blockers (used for treatment of high blood pressure) constrict air passages and thus are contraindicated in some pulmonary conditions. Cooling the airways may result in bronchial constriction, and exercise or hyperventilation in emotional stress may trigger asthmatic attacks, because of a lowering of the airway temperature.

The severity of asthma in a patient is judged by the presence of persistent airflow limitation, which puts asthma in a group of pulmonary conditions called Chronic Obstructive Pulmonary Diseases (or COPD).

COSMETICS AND ASTHMA

Symptom suggesting hyperreactivity of the respiratory tract and asthma provokes by perfume without the presence of bronchial obstruction.

Formaldehyde a toxic chemical used in industry in the manufacture of glues is also used as a preservative in cosmetics and for embalming bodies. Formaldehyde mixes easily with water but will not mix with oil or grease. It is common to find formaldehyde in aqueous cosmetic formulations such as shampoo; conditioner, shower gel, liquid hand wash and bubble bath; even products designed for children such as bubble bath and baby shampoo have formaldehyde in them.

Health effects of formaldehyde

Formaldehyde, a colourless, pungent-smelling gas, can cause watery eyes, burning sensations in the eyes and throat, nausea, and difficulty in breathing in some humans exposed at elevated levels (above 0.1 parts per million). High concentrations of formaldehyde may trigger asthma attacks in susceptible people.

The symptoms are not transmitted via the olfactory nerve, since the patients could not smell the perfume, but they may have been induced by a trigeminal reflex via the respiratory tract or by the eyes.

Perfume-scented strips in magazines can cause exacerbations of symptoms and airway obstruction in asthmatic patients.

Severe and atopic asthma increases risk of adverse respiratory reactions to perfumes.

ROLE OF POLLUTANTS

Asthma is related to air pollution. The human body does possess intricate protective mechanisms. The hair in the nasal cavity, acts as a barricade to inhaled dust particles. The mucus covering of the nasal and pharyngeal mucosa traps most of the air pollutants; hence throat clearing, nose blowing, and sneezing are more common in the presence of dusty air. These are natural protective reflexes that clear the load of polluting particles from the nose and throat and make this important barrier useful for protecting our lungs. Our tonsils, which consist of lymphatic tissue, are strategically positioned in the pharynx to assist the defense system of the upper respiratory tract. Constant exposure to pollutants, including bacteria and viruses that pass through the throat with air, drink and food renders the tonsils susceptible to infections. This fact often prompts surgical removal of tonsils, and this procedure, unfortunately, removes an important protective barrier against pollutants entering our body. We don't prefer this attempt as it is just like removing the soldiers from the border to invite the enemies (bacteria etc.) to enter freely.

Further down in the bronchial tree, the inhaled air is continuously screened and the presence of residual pollutants triggers the cough reflex initiated by a constriction of the air passages. This airway constriction facilitates slower airflow, preventing the polluted air from entering the alveoli (terminal structures in the lungs where the exchange of oxygen occurs). In response, we cough to force down the air (regardless of its quality) to the alveoli. This explains why coughing is not the healthy reflex of clearing something out of lungs, but rather a desperate attempt to breathe, which simultaneously forces the polluted air into the lungs. Coughing is therefore an important signal of distress from the lungs, very much like indigestion is a sign of distress from the digestive tract. Coughing along with sneezing often precedes an asthma attack and the related condition, "allergic rhinitis."

Fortunately, the polluting particles that sneak into the lower respiratory tract are flushed off by epithelial cilia (a microscopic hairlike structure) towards pharynx. These epithelial cells are covered with a layer of mucus, which traps the polluting particles and carries them out to the throat. But in an asthmatic patient due to a chronic inflammatory condition, the movement of ciliae is brought almost to a standstill, and the abnormally increased secretion of mucus makes airway passages obstructed for air that we breathe.

Another rapid reaction system in our lungs to counteract pollution is made of various immune cells (or body defence cells), which literally devour the foreign particles. These cells collectively are called white cells and by their function are referred to as macrophages - the cells that eat foreign matter. However, the action of white cells comes often at considerable cost to the airways themselves. When macrophages ingest large amounts of the substances contained in a cigarette smoke, or silica or asbestos particles of polluted air, they release enzymes (intended to digest the invader, i.e., antigen), which cause the inflammation of the airways and chronic, nagging cough. This is in fact a classic mechanism of a chronic inflammatory and degenerative condition of the bronchial tree, often referred to as bronchitis and too often initiating the deadly disease of emphysema. The current view of asthma is that it is "a chronic inflammatory disorder in which many white cells play a role, especially mast cells, eosinophils and T-lymphocytes".

CAUSES OF ASTHMA

Allergies

One cause of bronchial asthma is definitely allergic. An individual may have hay fever and asthma simultaneously during the ragweed season or may at this time experience attacks of asthma only. Other allergens may be responsible, including the dander from animal fur and feathers, face powder, or certain foods.

Infections

Many cases of bronchial asthma are associated with bacterial infections, especially of the sinuses, throat, and nose. Sometimes these improve very markedly when the infection clears up.

Nervous tension

Some cases of bronchial asthma appear to be due to nervous tension and often improve tremendously when the person's emotional problems are solved with the help of a counselor.

These cases become worse if the person is emotionally disturbed or tense. For this reason asthma is also included among the psychosomatic diseases.

Risk factors

The strongest risk factors for developing asthma are exposure, especially in infancy, to indoor allergens (such as domestic mites in bedding, carpets and stuffed furniture, cats and cockroaches) and a family history of asthma or allergy.

Exposure to tobacco smoke and exposure to chemical irritants in the workplace are additional risk factors. Other risk factors include certain drugs (aspirin and other non-steroid anti-inflammatory drugs), low birth weight and respiratory infection. The weather (cold air), extreme emotional expression and physical exercise can exacerbate asthma. Urbanization appears to be correlated with an increase in asthma.

PROVOKING FACTORS

Allergens

Inhaled e.g.: Dust, pollen, house dust, mite, sudden change in humidity level or sudden change in temperature like coming out from hot room or cold air condition etc.

Ingested e.g.: Fish, nuts, strawberries etc.

Food that trigger asthma

Food triggered asthma is unusual. Although food allergies may trigger asthma in a small number of people; not all individuals with food allergies have asthma. Substantial scientific investigation has found that the following foods and food additives can trigger asthma.

Some of the food allergens :

1. Milk
2. Eggs
3. Peanuts
4. Tree nuts
5. Soy
6. Wheat
7. Fish
8. Shellfish

Role of sulfites

Sulfites or sulfating agents, both occurring naturally or used in food processing, have been found to trigger asthma. If sulfites are used in food preparation or processing as a preservative agent, you will find them listed on the food label. Common food sources of sulfites include:

- Dried fruits or vegetables
- Potatoes (some packaged and prepared)
- Wine, beer
- Bottle lemon or lime juice
- Shrimp (fresh, frozen, or prepared)
- Pickled foods, such as pickles, relishes, peppers, or sauerkraut (some)

Sulfites and Sulphating agents : Sulphur dioxide, Sodium bisulfite, Potassium bisulfite, Sodium metabisulfite, Potassium metabisulfite, and Sodium sulfite.

Additives in food

1. Tatrazine yellow dye used as a colouring agent
2. Metabisulfite preservatives used in beers, wines and preserved foods.
3. Monosodium glutamate or "ajinomoto" added to Chinese food, which may precipitate asthma.

Other factors

1. Infections, mainly viral infections.
2. Environmental pollutants
3. Exercise
4. Emotions e.g., Laughing
5. Occupational allergens e.g., grain-dust, wood dust
6. Physio-chemical agents like gases, and smoke.

HISTOPATHOLOGY

A number of causes have been postulated for the increased airway reactivity of asthma. The most popular hypothesis at present is that of airway inflammation. Increased number of mast cells, neutrophils, eosinophils and lymphocytes has been found in the bronchoalveolar lavage fluids of patients with asthma as have a variety of mediators. An active inflammatory process is frequently observed in endo bronchial biopsy specimens even from asymptomatic patients. The cells that play important role are mast cells, eosinophils, macrophages, neutrophils and lymphocytes.

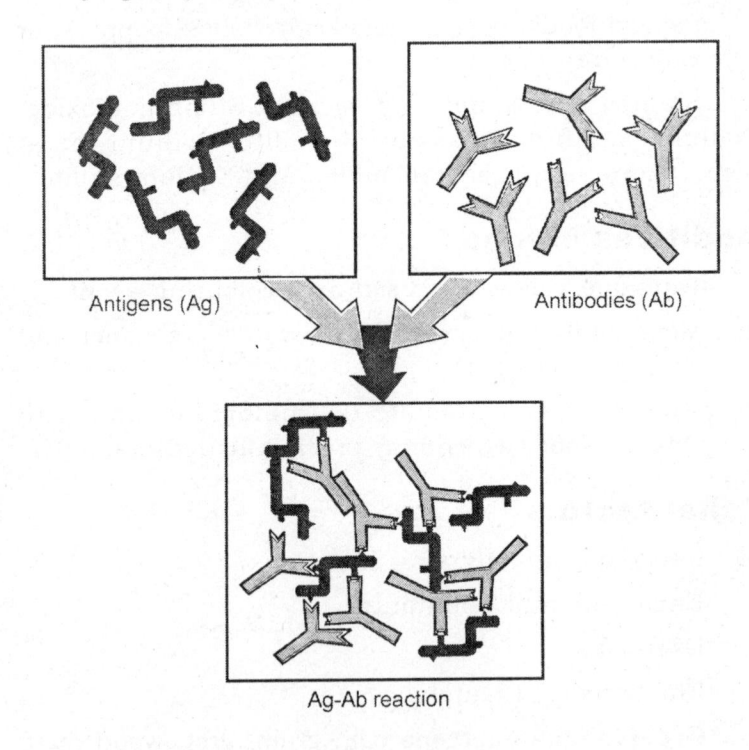

Antigens (Ag)

Antibodies (Ab)

Ag-Ab reaction

The antigen-antibody reaction is highly specific because the antibodies are tailor made for the antigen

The eosinophil appears to play an important part in the infiltrative component. The granular protein in this cell - major basic protein and eosinophilic cationic protein are capable of destroying the airway epithelium. T lymphocytes also appear to be important in the inflammatory response.

HOW DOES ASTHMA DEVELOP?

Allergen exposure

Atopic individuals are sensitised after an exposure to allergens and develop IgE antibodies. Subsequent exposure to allergen causes a dual response, which is protracted and more severe.

Early Asthmatic Response (EAR) (due to mast cell mediator release)	Late Asthmatic Response (LAR) (Due to T cell mediated influx or Inflammatory cells chiefly Eosinophils)
Reversible Obstructive Airway Disease (**ROAD**) (Bronchospasm)	Bronchial Hyper reactivity (**BHR**) (Inflammation)
Treated with Bronchodilators	Treated with anti inflammatory drugs.

Thus, asthma has two components:

ROAD (Bronchospasm), which can be reversed with broncho-dilators;

BHR due to inflammation (which predisposes to recurrent bronchospasm with minor stimuli like exercise, smoke, dust exposure, etc.) treated best with anti-inflammatory drugs.

This is a condition in which the small bronchial airways temporarily constrict, so that it is difficult to exhale. This leads to breathlessness and wheezing. Such difficulty is caused by muscle spasm in the bronchi of the lungs. This narrows the space available for air to make its way out of the lungs, and breathing out is always more difficult than breathing in, thus producing the characteristic wheezing sound associated with asthma attacks.

Because the passages are narrowed and airflow reduced, mucus also builds up in the lungs, and this makes it even more difficult to breathe. The mucus is also a breeding-ground for bacteria, so attacks of bronchitis may arise as a complication of the asthma.

A number of different groupings can be applied:

- **Extrinsic asthma** – caused by allergic responses to house dust, animal fur, or various foods. Such causes 10-20% of adult asthma.
- **Intrinsic asthma** – caused by genetics, structural problems, infections, pollutants and stress - both physiological and psychological. Such causes 30-50% of adult asthma.

The symptoms of people with asthma differ greatly in frequency and degree. Some have an occasional episode that is mild and brief; otherwise they are symptom free. Others have mild coughing and wheezing much of the time, punctuated by severe exacerbations of symptoms following exposure to known allergies, viral infections, and exercise or nonspecific irritants. A series of stages have been characterized for describing the severity of an acute asthma attack:

1. **Mild** — mild dyspnoea; diffuse wheezes; adequate air exchange.
2. **Moderate** — respiratory distress at rest; hyperapnoea, use of accessory muscles; marked wheezes.
3. **Severe** — marked respiratory distress; cyanosis; use of accessory muscles; marked wheezes or absent breathe sounds.
4. **Respiratory failure** — severe respiratory distress; lethargy; confusion; prominent pulsus paradoxus. Use of accessory muscles.

Irreversible airflow limitation

It is clearly established that irreversible airflow limitation develops in some asthma patients. This may be caused by increase of airway wall thickness due to accumulation of inflammatory cells, oedema, increased thickness of smooth muscle, sub-epithelial fibrosis and remodelling of the airway wall. Obstruction of the airway lumen by exudates and mucus, and changes of the elastic properties of the airway wall results in the loss of the interdependence between the airways and the surrounding parenchyma which contributes to the irreversible airflow. In most of the asthma patients, the hypertrophy of the smooth muscles is more pronounced in the central airways, but in a subgroup of patients, it also extends to peripheral bronchioles.

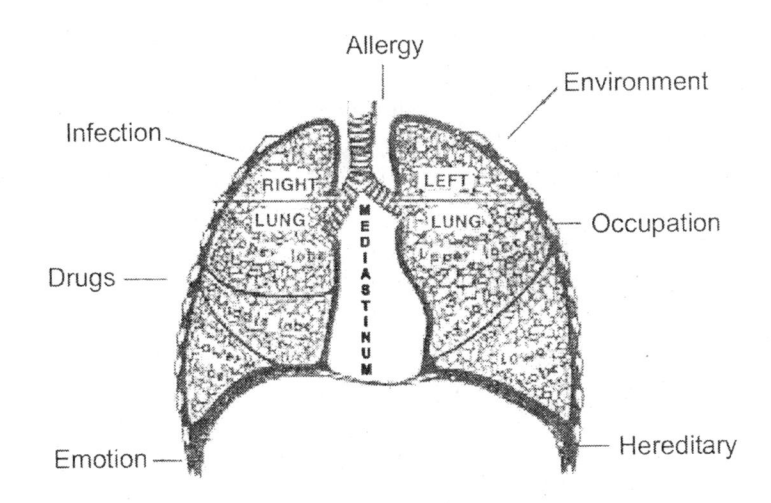

Bronchial Asthma : Modern Aetiology

Antigen antibody reaction

The role of mast cells in bronchial asthma :
Mast cells are pivotal in the allergic response type I or the anaphylactic type – a rapidly progressing chain-reaction that causes sudden attack of asthma. Mast cells are found around blood

vessels in the connective tissue, in the lining of the gut and importantly in the lining of the upper and lower respiratory tract. These are large mononuclear cells heavily granulated, with granules containing a host of pharmacologically active substances. The allergen (antigen) enters into the human body through the respiratory tract, skin and/or Gastro Intestinal Tract (GIT). After the exposure to antigens, antibodies directed against specific antigens. (i.e., IgE) are formed and are fixed to their respective receptors on the surface of the mast cells. This process is called sensitization of mast cells. During the second exposure to antigens, the antigens react with these antibodies at the cell surface. This event leads to a series of biochemical reactions. These migrate to the periphery in the secretory expulsion of the mast cell granules containing active substances (vasoactive amines and chemolytic amines) causing asthma attacks. This process is called "mast cell degranulation".

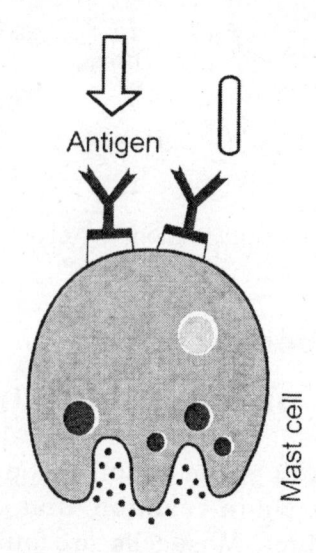

The role of epithelial cells in bronchial asthma : The central cell in the development of inflammation in airways are the mast cell. Also the epithelial cells which line the airway passages have a pivotal role in the initiation of allergic chain of events and in maintaining continuous inflammation.

The airway epithelium appears to be more than just a physical barrier protecting the integrity of airways. In many ways, it plays a role as a communicator sending its own messengers to the organism and requesting a response to the message. The substances synthesized and released by the epithelium in asthma syndrome are like the messengers responsible for attracting inflammatory cells to the airways. This chain of events contributes to the development of asthma syndrome.

The role of eosinophils in asthma : In asthma patients, the number of bronchial tree eosinophils in blood is increased during asthma attacks and tend to normalize once the patient becomes asymptomatic. Eosinophils are also considered to be the major inflammatory cells in asthma since these can damage the epithelial cells lining bronchial tree.

As soon as the eosinophils are established in the airways, they themselves, like other inflammatory cells, can produce messengers of inflammation, which in turn stimulate eosinophil production, and activation. Eosinophils play a crucial role in asthma because their presence sustains the inflammation in asthma. The nighttime worsening of asthma has been associated with the increase of eosinophils in the airways as well as increased presence of the chemical messengers of inflammation.

The role of T-cells in asthma development : The role of T lymphocytes in asthma syndrome can be described as regulatory or as that of a manager which regulates traffic of the inflammatory cells, specifically their arrival and departure as well inflammatory activity in the airways. The overall regulatory abilities of lymphocytes T are based mainly on existence of two specific subclasses of lympocytes T, i.e., T helper lymphocytes also known as CD4 which stimulate a particular immunological reaction (e.g. inflammation), and T suppressor lymphocytes also known as CD8+ which do the opposite, subduing the immunological reaction (e.g. inflammation). Upon exposure of the airways of the asthma patient to allergen CD4 T cells are being recruited from the blood and transferred to the airways.

Asthmatics in comparison to healthy individuals show an elevated percentage of CD4 cells in the airways. In asthmatics, the percentage of CD4 cells correlate positively with the severity of the condition as well as the number of blood eosinophils.

The CD4, but not CD8 lymphocytes from asthmatics, may be helping in the eosinophil survival. This is how CD4 T lymphocytes regulate inflammation in asthma, and also make the therapeutic approaches clear in asthma.

Prognosis

Allergic rhinitis is easily treatable but relapse is very common because of unhindered access of allergens through air. Even patients with 'controlled' asthma get frequent relapses of AR, which has been termed as 'reversion'. This appears quickly during a comprehensive therapy for bronchial asthma alone, while AR remains untreated.

The frequent relapse of AR is due to the steady and unhindered access of allergens in the nasal cavity. Nasal hairs (vibrissae), sticky mucus over the nasal epithelium, ciliated movements, nasal secretary IgA and protective reflexes of sneezing, warming and moistening of the air are some of the ways by which outside air with allergens are contained. The same air then reaches the LRT, devoid of many of the harmful agents. Nasal stimuli like soluble allergens or histamine and methacholine may become absorbed through nasal mucosa and cause both AR and BHR (Bronchial hyperreactivity).

ASTHMA AND SKIN DISEASES

Early onset Asthma occurs in atopic individuals i.e. those who readily form allergenic antibodies to commonly encountered allergens. As a result they get various skin disorders. Such individuals can be identified by skin sensitivity test, which give positive reactions with a wide range of common allergens.

Atopic dermatitis is a chronic or recurrent atopic inflammatory skin disease that usually begins in the first few years of life. It is often the initial clinical manifestation of an atopic predisposition and often precedes allergic rhinitis and asthma in children. It may be present at any age, but usually has an onset in infancy. It may be associated with allergy.

SEASON AND ASTHMA

Episodic Asthma are usually worse in the summer, when they are more heavily exposed to antigens, while chronic Asthmaticus are usually worse in the winter month because of their increased liability to bacterial infection.

Spring, with all its airborne pollen, is the cruellest season for asthma and allergy sufferers. Spring brings warm days, gentle rains, and high pollen counts — and, in the case of about one person in five, a miserable siege of hay fever.

Allergies can happen any time of year, but spring, with its exuberant burst of plant life, fills the air with wind-borne pollen. In people with hay fever, the pollen is an allergen, which prompts the immune system to produce an antibody called IGE, which attaches to what are known as mast cells. The mast cells release histamines and other chemicals that make the nose run, cause repeated sneezing, and set the eyes, nose, ears, and throat to itching — the typical hay fever symptoms.

PREGNANCY AND ASTHMA

Asthma is a common obstructive pulmonary disease during the childbearing age. It occurs in 0.4% to 1.3% of pregnant patients.

An increased responsiveness of the tracheo-bronchial tree to various stimuli leads to bronchoconstriction. Widespread narrowing of small and large airways, along with excessive production of thick mucus, causes airway plugging. Attacks can abate spontaneously or as a result of therapy. The clinical manifestations are paroxysms of dyspnoea, cough and wheezing of various degrees (mild to severe).

TYPES OF ASTHMA

The Seasonal Type — If the patient's asthma always returns with a certain season of the year, it is obviously due to something that he smells or eats at that time alone. The usual and very common cause is the grass pollen. Patients may have pure asthma from this cause without the usual symptoms of hay fever, though such an occurrence is rare.

The Locality Type — Patients have been known to

lose their asthma by going to live on the opposite side of a road or even by sleeping in a different room in their own home. Many of these cases are explained by the fact that an animal has been left behind, or some ivy or creeper avoided that previously gave rise to asthma symptoms. Many complain that they cannot stand the sea.

The Periodic Type — A few cases seem to show an extraordinarily regular periodicity of onset. Every fourteen or fifteen days an attack comes, without any regard to specific days of the week. It seems as though such cases are desensitised by an attack; when the desensitisation has gradually worked off, they again become sensitive and have another attack.

The Menstrual Type — Many patients date the commencement of their asthma from the time of puberty, and many women have exacerbations of asthma at the menstrual periods regularly throughout their life. As in many other menstrual disturbances, this may be during the week before the period commencement or during its flow. This opens up the question of the endocrine glands and their influence in asthma and its allied complaints.

The Occupation Type — This type merely consists of those patients who are sensitive to proteins they meet with at their work. Many are also examples of cases, which become sensitive only after very long years of work at one particular occupation. Such patients could be poultry keepers, farmers, ostlers, and bakers.

CONSEQUENCE OF SLEEP ON RESPIRATORY MUSCLES

There is decrease in lung ventilation during sleep and upper airway resistance increases especially during REM.

More respiratory efforts can lead to snoring and even upper airway collapse.

As in Orthopnoea we observe the difficulty in breathing in lying position. This dyspnoea on lying flat is relieved by sitting up.

Orthopnoea occurs when right atrial and right ventricular function is relatively normal but there is impaired function on the left side of the heart.

In supine position there is an increase in venous return to the right atrium and the right ventricle, and hence an increase in blood flow to the lungs.

Effects of sleep on the control of breathing

Sleep is associated with overall reductions in lung ventilation compared to waking.

Decreases in tidal volume importantly contribute to the decreased ventilation. Decreases in respiratory rate occur less consistently in sleeping humans, although respiratory slowing does occur in some individual.

Decrease in tidal volume and lung ventilation occur in sleep because of changes in the control of breathing in sleep:

1. Decreased activation of respiratory muscles.
2. Increased upper airway resistance.
3. Reduced compensatory responses to this respiratory load.
4. An increase in the level of arterial CO_2 required to maintain spontaneous breathing.
5. Reduced ventilator responses to the increased CO_2.
6. Little effect due to changes in ventilator responses to O_2.

DIAGNOSIS

A diagnosis of asthma should be considered if the following features are present:

History

Presence of atopy i.e. history of asthma, allergic rhinitis, atopic dermatitis, eczema or urticaria in any of the family members.

Dyspnoea with wheezing, which may be episodic initially and continuous later.

Unexplained cough with or without viscid sputum.

Past diagnosis of frequent "allergic bronchitis", "asthmatic bronchitis" or "eosinophilla".

Physical examination

1. General: Tachypnoea, tachycardia, use of accessory muscles of respiration, subcostal or intercostals retraction (These are signs of acute episodic attack of asthma).
2. Lungs: Since asthmatic symptoms are variable through the day, the physical examination of the respiratory system may appear normal. The combination of hyperinflation and advanced airflow limitation in an asthma exacerbation also markedly increases the work of breathing.

Clinical signs of dyspnoea

- Prolonged expiratory phase associated with wheezing and hyperinflation is more likely to be present if patients are examined during symptomatic periods and in the morning prior to the administration of a bronchodilator. Wheezing sound is caused by passage of the air current through bronchi narrowed by exudates.
- Sonorous and sibilant rhonchi: musical or wheezing sound when produced in the large bronchi with a deep toned note is sonorous rhonchi. When arising in smallest bronchi with a high pitched squeak its sibilant rhonchi.

Rhonchi are often more consipicious during expiration because then the bronchi are normally narrower than during inspiration and they are vesicular in character.

- In a severe attack cyanosis may also be seen. Cyanosis is a blue discolouration of the skin or mucosa and is usually a sign of severe oxygen deficiency. It is of central type in Asthma due to deficient oxygenation of blood in the lungs resulting from inadequate ventilation of perfused areas of lung.
- The percussion note may be hyper resonant.
- Clubbing of fingers may be present when Asthma occurs as a complication of or is associated with bronchiectasis and bronchial carcinoma.

Investigation

1. Normal chest radiogram, which may show enhanced vascular markings.
2. Peripheral smear showing Eosinophilia.
3. Pulmonary function test: low FEV/ FVC ratio.

FVC= The maximum amount of air forcefully expired after maximum inspiration

FEV = The amount of air forcefully expired in the first second of an FVC

GRADING SCALE FOR DYSPNOEA

An affirmative answer to one of the following questions establishes a patient's grade:

Grade I : "Are you ever troubled by breathlessness, other than on strenuous exertion?"

Grade II : "Are you short of breath when hurrying on level ground or walking up a slight hill?"

Grade III : "Do you have to walk slower than most people on level ground? Do you have to stop after a mile or so (or after 15 minutes) when you walk on level ground at your own pace?"

Grade IV : "Do you have to stop for breath after walking about 100 yards (or after a few minutes) on level ground?"

Grade V : "Are you too breathless to leave the house or breathless after undressing?"

MANAGEMENT

- Control symptoms so as to maintain normal activity levels, including exercise.
- Maintain pulmonary function as close to the normal levels as possible.
- Avoid or control asthma triggering factors.
- Establish plans for the prevention and manage-ment of exacerbations.

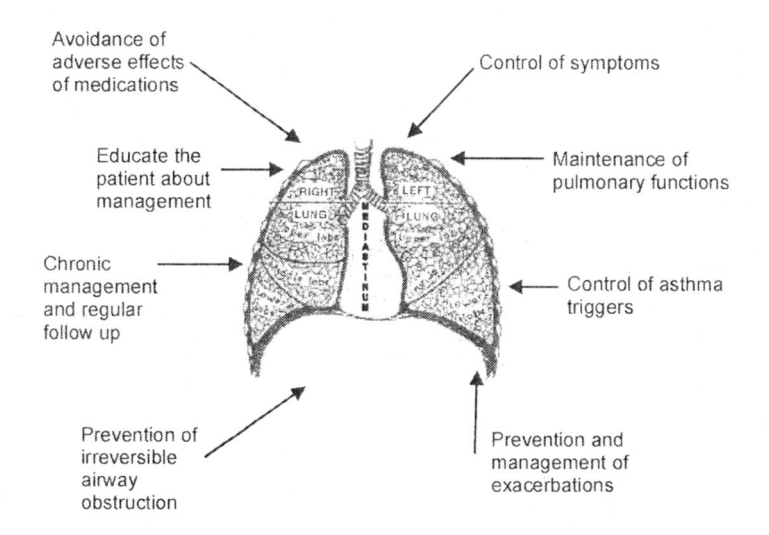

Asthma Management

- Avoid adverse affects from asthma medications.
- Educate patients to develop a partnership in asthma management.
- Establish plans for chronic management and regular follow up.

Prevent development of irreversible airway obstruction and reduce asthma mortality by strict adherence to the above goals.

4

AYURVEDIC CONCEPT

In Ayurveda, the exact causes for asthma are fully described which are mainly related to dietary habits, way of life, environment and constitution of the body. On the other hand, modern science considers allergic substances to be responsible for the causation of asthma. But, not all persons who are exposed to allergens, suffer from the disease, it is only few who react towards them. The question arises then, what causes this selectivity, why do some suffer and others don't?

In Ayurveda, the basic concept is that of Tridosha–Vata, Pitta and Kapha. An individual's body is composed of seven categories of fundamental tissue elements: malas - waste products of the body produced at the end of digestive and metabolic processes. Functioning of the entire body is regulated by the three doshas. In a healthy person, all these three types of elements are in a state of equilibrium. When the equilibrium is disturbed, it results in ill health. External factors, sensory influences, and foodstuffs influence these three elements, Tridoshas. Hence, according to Ayurveda, allergy is not the primary cause of the disease but a precipitating factor, which attack the person whose Tridoshas are already in the state of disequilibrium. Before going into a detailed description of asthma according to Ayurveda, we should discuss some basic concepts of Ayurveda.

Ayurveda believes that 'sum dosha – sum dhatu and sum agni' develop strong immune system. It states that 'Mithya Ahar – Vihar' i.e. wrong eating habits, pollution, infections, mental stress and moist atmosphere decrease the immunity and weaken the defence system of the body which effect 'shwasprashwas Tantra' and cause asthma.

THE TRIDOSHA CONCEPT

All matter is built on the basis of the 'Mahabhutas' or building blocks of existence, but only living matter has the Tridoshas, the three forces regulating all biological processes. They arise out of the basic elements and are treated in Ayurvedic literature as substances although they are not. They are dynamic principles, three different form of energy, which govern the entire energy reserves in the living organisms. From the simplest activity in a cell to the most complicated bodily function, the Tridoshas permit and control everything that is going on. They always work as a team and one never appears disharmony, decides the objective condition of a living being. A harmonious relationship of the three-bioenergetics principles is the mark of good health. Any imbalance, the equilibrium becomes unstable and reveals itself in a wide variety of symptoms.

The vata doshas and its five divisions

Of the three doshas, vata is the most important, since it sets the other two doshas in motion. It is responsible for all the body's sensations and activities. Perception, assimilation, and reaction are all properties of Vata, which channelise the perceptions through the sense organs, transform them into psychic events, and produce an appropriate reaction via the executive organs. Vata converts everything experienced by the senses into psychosomatic reactions, and thus is often equated with the vital force or vitality. It animates the psyche, regulates the breathing and creates activity. Even the two other dosha receive their motive energy from Vata.

Following is a comparative table of the features of a well-balanced vata (physiological vata) and of a disordered vata (pathological vata).

Vata

Physiological (Normal Function)	Pathological (Disturbed Function)
1. Proper regulation of all the body's activities.	1. The body's activities are impaired, upset & inhibited.
2. Fit for conception.	2. Unfit for conception.
3. Healthy development of the foetus. Natural parturition.	3. Malformation or miscarriage of foetus. Uterine inertia.
4. Normal initiation of the movement of eating, digestion and excretion.	4. The movements for eating, digestion and excretion are disturbed or even paralysed.
5. Mental activity. Control & guidance of mental processes.	5. Mental inactivity, confusion and memory impaired.
6. Good control of the organs of perception and of the reactions of the executive organs.	6. The normal function of perception and reaction are disturbed. Dullness of senses and slowing of responses.
7. Stimulation of digestion and the secretion of gastric and other digestive juices.	7. Deficient secretion of gastric and other digestive juices.
8. Initiation of the wish and will to lead an active life. Imparts vitality and natural excitation.	8. Loss of energy and the joy of living or over excitement.
9. Drying up of excessive and pathological discharges provoked by the other two Doshas.	9. Pathological discharges due to an imbalanced state of the other two Doshas are no longer dried up and combated.
10. Keeping the breathing regular and in a normal manner.	10. Respiratory disorders.
11. Reinforcement in the life; promotion of longevity.	11. Obstruction of the life flow; shortening of life.

Ayurveda divides this biogenic force "Vata" which has so many diverse functions, into five subsidiary forms differing from one another by their localization in the body and by their particular functions, although together they make the "power of vata". They are Prana, Udana, Vyana, Samana and Apana.

1. Prana (life force): It is located in the heart, brain and the chest. It controls the breathing, the mind, the senses and sustains the heart.
2. Udana (rising air): It is located in the thorax and nose. It controls speech, memory and intellect.
3. Samana (associated with digestive fire): It is located in the stomach and small intestines. It controls digestion and the secretion of gastric juices.
4. Apana (downward breath): It is located in the colon and pelvic organs and controls elimi-nation of stool, urine, semen and menstrual fluid.
5. Vyana (Diffused throughout the body): It is located in the heart. It controls the functioning of the circulatory channels like blood vessels.

The pitta dosha and its five divisions

The principle Pitta, belongs to every reaction, have a heating factor, which is either generated or utilized. Its main function is transformation of food in the body and in all metabolic processes. Pitta has the energy of the element fire, to create warmth, and to be vivid and restless. Pitta is known as the impetus of life; it stimulates the intellect and the capacity of enthusiasm and encourages singleness of the mind.

The following is a comparative table of the features of a well balanced and an unbalanced Pitta.

Pitta

Physiological (Normal Function)	Pathological (Disturbed Function)
1. Activation and regulation of the digestion.	1. Poor digestion. Imperfect separation of nutrients and waste materials.
2. Preserves the vision.	2. Impaired vision.
3. Regulates body temperature.	3. Body temperature, unregulated.
4. Definite skin colour. Normal appearance and lustre.	4. Dull appearance. Various skin colours.
5. Courage.	5. Anxiety.
6. A happy disposition.	6. Irritability dominates.
7. Colours the blood, normal blood haemoglobin.	7. A deficiency of haemoglobin.
8. Promotes intellectual capacity.	8. Mental apathy, deficient intelligence.
9. Absorb substances smeared on the skin.	9. Reduced absorbency of the skin.
10. High ideals, striving for real value.	10. Spiritual poverty.

The "Power of Fire", like the "Power of Wind" is divided into five varieties: Alochaka, Pachaka, Ranjaka, Sadhaka and Bhrajaka, taken together they represent the force known as Pitta.

1. Pachaka (Digestion): It is located in the stomach and intestines and controls digestions.

2. Ranjaka (Colouring matter): It is located in the liver and spleen and controls red blood cor-puscles formations.

3. Sadhaka (Faculty of efficiency): It is located in the heart and controls memory and other related functions.

4. Alochaka (Faculty of vision): It is located in the eyes and helps in maintaining normal sight.

5. Bhrajaka (Shine): It is located in the skin. Bhrajaka colours and blazes the skin.

The kapha dosha and its five divisions

The principle Kapha, is a formative force. It provides particular dimensions of specific shapes to everything from an individual cell to the skeletal frame: it lends strength and stability and also makes the body supple. It provides mental and physical strength, stability and endurance. Putting on weight is also a result of Kapha. This principle can accelerate the healing process and can build up resistance against disease. Generally speaking wherever the effects of Vata and Pitta are seen in the body, Kapha keeps these two forces confined within their natural limits. Without the power of Kapha, the material universe would be as formless as wind and fire and would have no cohesion without Shleshma (a synonym of Kapha, in Sanskrit means, "cementing" or "cohering"). Kapha provides the body with stability, firmness, flexibility, resilience, coolness and media for the interplay of energetic or stimulating biogenic forces.

The following table lists the properties of harmonious and inharmonious Kapha.

Kapha

	Physiological (Normal Function)		Pathological (Disturbed Function)
1.	Moistness and lubricates.	1.	Asynovia, and under production of mucus in the digestive tract and of saliva.
2.	Firmness of joints.	2.	Loose joints.
3.	Hardness, stability and compactness.	3.	Looseness, instability and porosity.
4.	Strength of character and determination.	4.	Instability, weakness and laziness.
5.	Seriousness of intent.	5.	Gives up easily.
6.	Plumpness, firm muscle tone and a good state of nutrition.	6.	Emaciation, poor state of nutrition.
7.	Sexual potency.	7.	Impotence.
8.	Physical strength.	8.	Physical weakness.
9.	Willingness to forgive.	9.	Intolerance, revengeful, Discontent.
10.	Freedom from envy.	10.	Envy and jealousy.

The many operations of the force Kapha, which extends from the body's most important functions, far into the mental and character-building regions, Tarpaka and Sleshaka Kapha differ in their locations and functions, but together they comprise the force Kapha.

1. Kledaka (Moistens): It is located in the stomach. It moistens the food, thereby helping digestion.
2. Avalambaka (Supports): It is located in the heart and lungs and controls their functioning.
3. Bodhaka (Perception): It is located in the tongue. It controls the perception of taste.
4. Tarpaka (Faculty of satisfaction): It is located in the head and nourishes and performs its lubrication.
5. Shleshaka (Faculty of connection): It is located in the joints and performs its lubrication.

The Tridoshas, the functional units of the body, also determine, according to their relative strengths, the constitutional types of temperaments. They mould the basic character of an individual. People from each of the three psychosomatic character types differ from one another in state of health, in susceptibility to certain diseases, and in their response to medication, e.g. with an allergic reaction. They also differ in their emotions, in the way their minds work, and in their handling of external conditions.

This is where Ayurvedic diagnosis, which looks at the whole man, is able to score, based on its knowledge of Tridoshas and their disturbances. Therapy, too, is holistic; guided by the same condition of the doshas.

NATURAL URGES

In the Ayurvedic text, "Charaka Samhita", 13 types of natural urges are mentioned. According to Ayurveda urges should not be suppressed; otherwise various diseases may result. When the urges are not controlled or discharged properly, mental tension and conflicts may arise and various psychosomatic and psychiatric illnesses may result. Vata manifests natural urges in an individual. It is the reaction of the body to throw out the undesirable waste products. The following are the 13 natural urges :

1. Urge for micturition
2. Urge for defaecation
3. Urge for seminal ejaculation
4. Urge for flatus

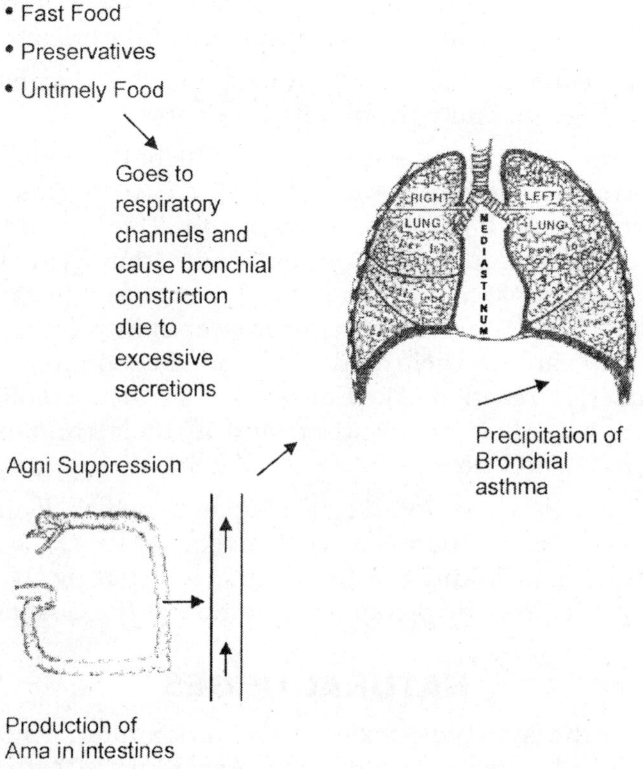

- Fast Food
- Preservatives
- Untimely Food

Goes to respiratory channels and cause bronchial constriction due to excessive secretions

Precipitation of Bronchial asthma

Agni Suppression

Production of Ama in intestines

Bronchial Asthma : The Ayurveda View

5. Urge for vomiting
6. Urge for sneezing
7. Urge for eructation
8. Urge for yawning
9. Urge for hunger
10. Urge for thirst
11. Urge for tears
12. Urge for sleep
13. Urge for breathing

Vata is involved in the manifestation of these urges; it controls the functioning of lungs and the rest of the respiratory system. Therefore if urges are suppressed it leads to vitiation of Vata, which can further give rise to number of diseases including asthma.

THE CONCEPT OF SAPTA DHATU (SEVEN BODY TISSUES)

The dhatus are the building blocks or fundamental tissues of the body. The seven fundamental tissues are:

Rasa	Body fluids/ plasma, lymph.
Rakta	Blood cells
Mamsa	Muscular tissues/muscles, dense or collagenous, elastic, reticular etc.
Meda	Adipose tissue/ fat
Asthi	Bone (osseous)/cartilagenous or chondrocytes
Majja	Nerve tissue/ bone marrow
Shukra	Generative tissue/semen

The meaning of "dhatu" is to support and to nourish. They support the body individually and collectively by performing their normal functions and they nourish the doshas, following them. The anatomy and physiology of dhatu in Ayurveda is explained in great detail but here, from the point of view of understanding either pathogenesis of the disease, or maintenance of health, it would suffice to know that these dhatus exist in a particular order of importance relative to each other.

It is envisaged that dietary constituents, after undergoing digestion (leading to the formation of normal digestive product rasa; metabolic products; vipaka or abnormal products; ama) are assimilated in the Rasadhatu first. This then distributes, to various tissues (dhatus) to nourish them. The way of distribution is sequential. Thus, shukradhatu is the last to receive nutrients.

In this way, all the dhatus receive nutrient from the Rasadhatu. Specific nutrient is picked up by specific "srotas" of the respective dhatus according to their requirement and availability.

In this manner nourishment and rebuilding of the supporting tissues of the body (dhatus) takes place.

MALAS

Mala are conventionally interpreted as excretory products. However, they are products of digestion of food as well as cellular metabolism, and are not always harmful and often play a protective role. Therefore, mala can be more appropriately interpreted as metabolic end products rather than excretory products.

SROTAS

The following 13 types of srotas are mentioned
1. Prana Vaha Srotas
2. Udaka Vaha Srotas
3. Anna Vaha Srotas
4. Rasa Vaha Srotas

5. Rakta Vaha Srotas

6. Mamsa Vaha Srotas

7. Medo Vaha Srotas

8. Asthi Vaha Srotas

9. Majja Vaha Srotas

10. Shukra Vaha Srotas

11. Mutra Vaha Srotas

12. Purisha Vaha Srotas

13. Sveda Vaha Srotas

THE CONCEPT OF SROTAS

Srotas are considered to be vast and complex transport systems of the body.

The substances, which nourish the dhatu, are made available to them through their own specific srotas, which are called as dhatuvaha srotas. Dhatuvaha srotas possesses a selective discrimination as to the kind of nutrients that should be made available to the respective dhatus and dhatu also exhibits a corresponding discriminating affinity for the kind of nutrition they need.

The srotas are innumerable and diverse (as are the elements that compose the body structure. Srotas spread through the body and nourish the different dhatus. No structure in the body can grow and develop independent of the srotas. When the integrity of the srotas is impaired, the dhatu is impaired, and vice verse. Morbidity spread from one dhatu to the other and from one srotas to the other because of their interdependence.

Impairment of the functional integrity of srotas, leads to its inability to perform normal functions resulting in the impairment of the function of the dhatu (or element related to that srotas). For example the Pranvaha srotas, when diseased, leads to difficulty in breathing. While if

Annavaha srotas is vitiated, they allow ama (which are undigested macromolecules of food) to pass into Rasadhatu and as a result of pathogenesis, the disease may take place in any system or organ depending upon the pressure of Khavaigunya (compromised function) at that particular site.

Root of Pranavaha Srotas : The origin of this srotas is Heart and food carrying channel (Annavahini dhamni).

This srotas carry vitality and vital breath.

They are vitiated by wasting, suppression of natural urges, intake of innutritious food, etc.

The signs of their vitiation are prolonged, restricted, shallow and frequent breathing.

The pathology of Asthma involves the concept of Agni and the concept of Ama along with the Pranavaha srotas vitiation.

CONCEPT OF AGNI

The term Agni comprehends various factors, which direct and participate in the course of digestion and metabolism in a living organism. Agni denotes digestion & metabolism in the body, which also includes neutralization of some toxic substances ingested by us. Hence, with a good status of Agni in the body, proper utilisation of food, detoxification of harmful substances etc. can take place which increases the body's resistance power by augmenting cellular functions. This is evident from the fact that different people taking the same kind of diet, exposed to the same environment, show selectivity in their reaction towards allergens/ etiological factors of the disease. Thus, Agni being one of the major factors responsible for this variation in response to stimuli is of vital importance in the state of health as well as in manifestation of disease.

CONCEPT OF AMA

The relationship between the endogenous and exogenous factors causing diseases is exemplified by the concept of ama. Ama is considered to be a product of improper assimilation of dietary constituents. "Improper assimilation or formation of intermediate products of digestion have toxic properties and are treated as foreign compounds by the body". Ama, results from the hypo function of Agni, the term relating to both pachakagni (digestive enzymes) and dhatvagni (metabolic enzymes). Ama and the interaction caused by ama with doshadhatu mala are considered to be toxic to the body. In fact ama is considered "poisonous or poison."

Ama, through the blood, reaches the respiratory channels and causes constriction or spasm of the alveoli, resulting in Asthma. Thus apart from clearing the bowel, it is also necessary to remove these waste products from the body.

GENERAL CAUSES OF ASTHMA

1. According to Ayurveda, Shvasa Roga (asthma) is caused by the vitiation of Vata and Kapha doshas. So, causes for vitiation of Vata and Kapha are also the causes for asthma.
2. Causes of vitiations of Vata: Cold water, excessive exercise, fasting, weakness, intake of dry food, suppression of natural urges, inhalation of dust and smoke, excessive intercourse etc.
3. Causes of vitiation of Kapha: Intake of excessive and heavy, oily food, use of curd, meat of aquatic animals especially seafood, and sesame oil.
4. Other diseases causing asthma: In Anaemia, diarrhoea, fever, vomiting, rhinitis, tuberculosis and scurvy, asthma is taken as a symptom. In heart disease, ascitis, gout, cirrhosis of liver and kidney disorders, asthma is taken as a secondary symptom.

VYADHI (DISEASE) TYPE

Asthma falls in following two types of vyadhi classification :

1. Kalbalpravritta – Seasonal Asthma

This group includes diseases, which are caused by Meteorological changes, like changes in the atmospheric temperature – hot or cold – humidity or dryness, rain and wind, incidental to changes in the season.

These diseases can be classified under two sub-heads, according to the seasons, which changes and exhibit either their natural or normal trait or abnormal, sub-normal or perverse traits. The former is responsible for the causation of disorders arising out of the usual adaptive reactions of the body. They are known as avyapannartu-krita vyadhis. The latter-vyapannartu-krita diseases consequent on the inability of the body to adapt itself to sudden and abnormal climatic and seasonal variations. Thus asthma falls in this category of vyapannartu krita vyadhi.

"Kalbalpravrita ye sheetoshne vata varsha tapa prabhriti nimitah teapi dwidhaVyapannaritukritah; avyapannaritukritasch."

2. Janmabal pravritta

The kind of diseases included under this category comprise of congenital types. Atopic types of Asthma fall in this category.

TYPE OF ASTHMA

1. Maha Shvasa (Biot's respiration).
2. Urdhva Shvasa (Stertorous breathing or respiratory failure).

3. Chinna Shvasa (Chyne stokes respiration).
4. Tamaka Shvasa (Bronchial asthma).
5. Kshudra Shvasa (Minor types of asthma, exertional dyspnoea).

THE SUMMARY OF THE CONCEPT OF DOSHA-DHATU-MALA

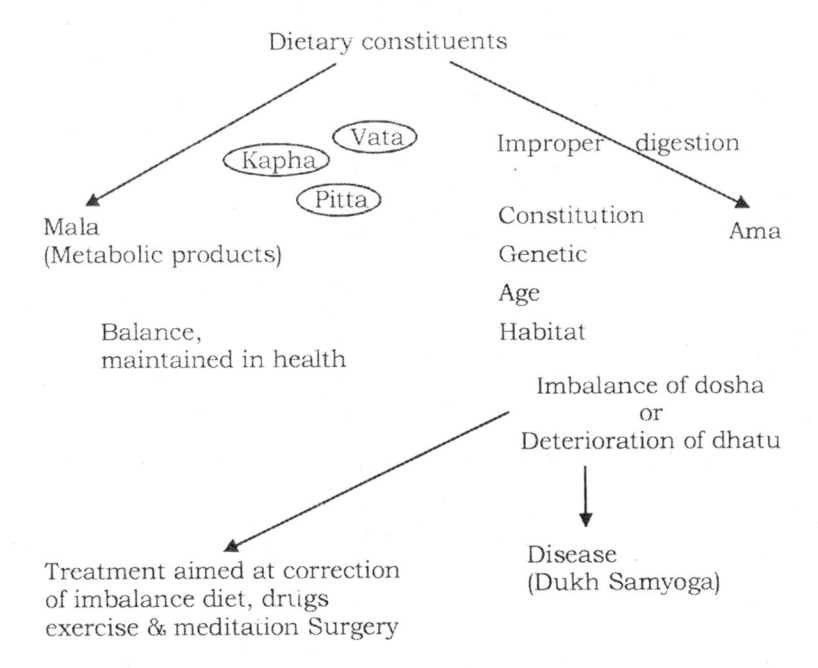

Dietary constituents

Kapha, Vata, Pitta

Mala (Metabolic products)

Improper digestion

Constitution
Genetic
Age
Habitat

Ama

Balance, maintained in health

Imbalance of dosha
or
Deterioration of dhatu

↓

Treatment aimed at correction of imbalance diet, drugs exercise & meditation Surgery

Disease
(Dukh Samyoga)

Applied aspect of dosha-dhatu-mala-concept

The derangement of dosha-dhatu-mala in the first place gives rise to dosha dushti (disease processes) and to dhatu dushti resulting in diseased structure and finally sthana dushti – dysfunction of organ.

The intricate interrelationship between the different functional units, stress on the role played by diet and other apparently harmless environmental factors in altering the dosha, mala and srotas and subsequently causing disease, as shown here:

Causation of disease

```
                    Causation of Diseases
                         Ahara
                         |
                         Rasadhatu
                                        Mala, dosha
   Ama

                              Srota
   Indirect                   dhatu
                         genetic
                         constitution ——▶ Disease
                              ▲
                              |
                         Direct
```

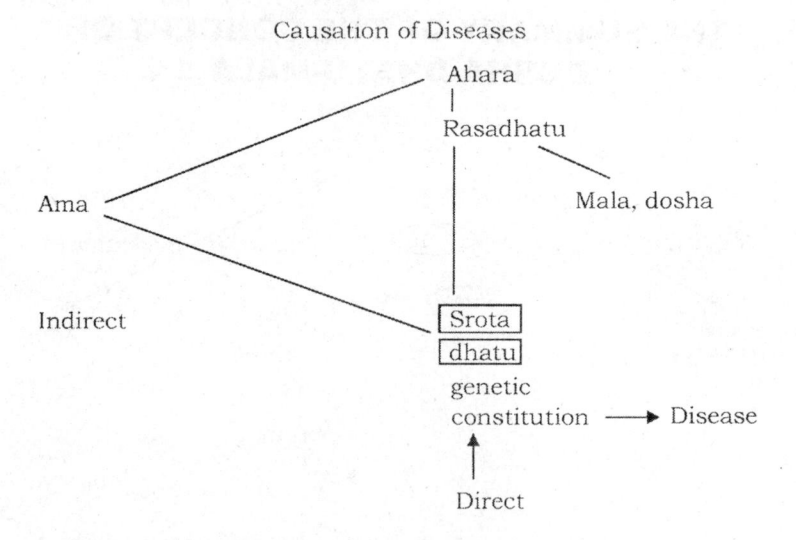

Congenital susceptibility or External/ Internal Stress

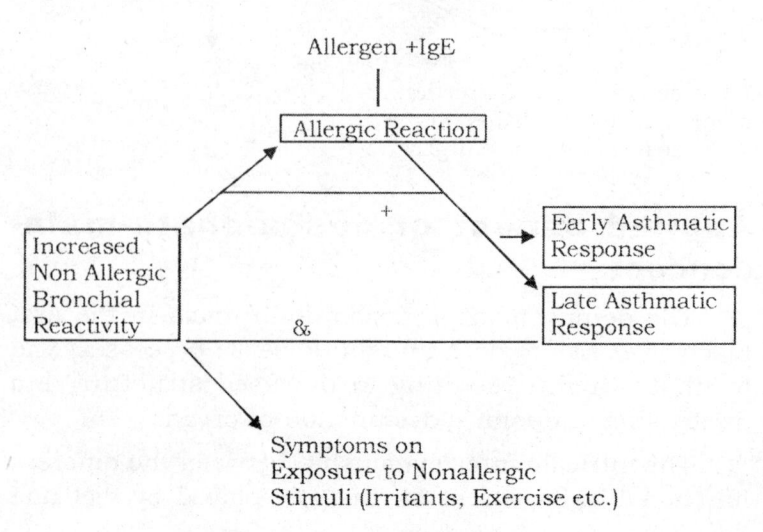

```
                    Allergen +IgE
                         |
                    Allergic Reaction
                    ↗           ↘
                        +          Early Asthmatic
  Increased                        Response
  Non Allergic
  Bronchial                        Late Asthmatic
  Reactivity       &                Response
       ↓
   Symptoms on
   Exposure to Nonallergic
   Stimuli (Irritants, Exercise etc.)
```

This ray diagram shows the relationship of the acute allergic reaction to the late asthmatic response and to bronchial hyper-reactivity; Airway hyper responsiveness and late asthmatic response.

PATHOLOGY OF ASTHMA (SAMPRATI)

"Yada srotansi sannrudhya marutah kaphapurvakha Vishvagvrajti sanrudhstatha shwasan karoti saha"

(Su. U. 51)

Asthma originates in the stomach. (The seat of Agni) passes through channels carrying rasa and gets located in the lungs.

Vitiation of Kapha : It causes anorexia and formation of ama leading to obstruction causing excessive secretion of Kapha (tenacious mucus). This excessive mucus leads to the obstruction of Pranavaha srotas, which is also aggravated due to inflammation of bronchioles caused by Kapha and Vata.

Vitiation of Vata : It causes obstruction of Pranavaha srotas leading to asthma due to spasm and inflammation in bronchioles caused by Vata.

Dosha : Vata and Kapha

Dushya : Rasa

Srotas : Pranvahasrotas

Dushti Lakshan :

"Atisrashtam Atibadham Kupitalpabhikshanam Vashabda Sashooluchvasantam......."

Frequent and shallow breathing, prolonged and restricted breath accompanied by abnormal respiratory sounds and pain.

Rasavasrotas and Pranavahasrotas are also involved

Origin: Stomach (Pitta sthana).

AVRAN

All the activities of the body are governed by vayu but when the quantity of toxins, doshas, dhatu, mala increases in the body they tend to overlap the physiological functioning of vayu which gives rise to pathological conditions of AVRAN.

E.g. When Sun is covered by the clouds, which are formed due to increased humidity in the atmosphere; result is diminished sunlight.

1. As mentioned earlier the foetus doesn't cry as the throat is full of KAPHA and sound-producing air passage is blocked, this Kapha is enveloping the udana vayu or obstructing the passage of vayu, the condition is similar to the samprapti of Asthma.

   "Jarayuna mukhechhine kanthe cha kaphaveshtite;
   Vayormargnirodhach na garbhasthah praroditi."

   Sushrut sharir sthan 2/54

   At birth the alveoli of a baby are so completely collapsed that a pressure difference of as much as 30 mmHg is required to expand them for the first time. Thus the first breath of life requires an extra ordinary effort to overcome the surface tension of the wall.

2. Prana Avritta Udana – Asthma is one of the symptoms of the pathological condition where prana vayu envelops udana. Charak in the chikitsa part prefers nasyam & dhumpan in this case.

3. Udana Avritta Apana - Shwasa is also a feature when udana vayu covers the Apana. Charaka advises vasti and food regime, which regulates vayu for this condition.

Samprapti chart

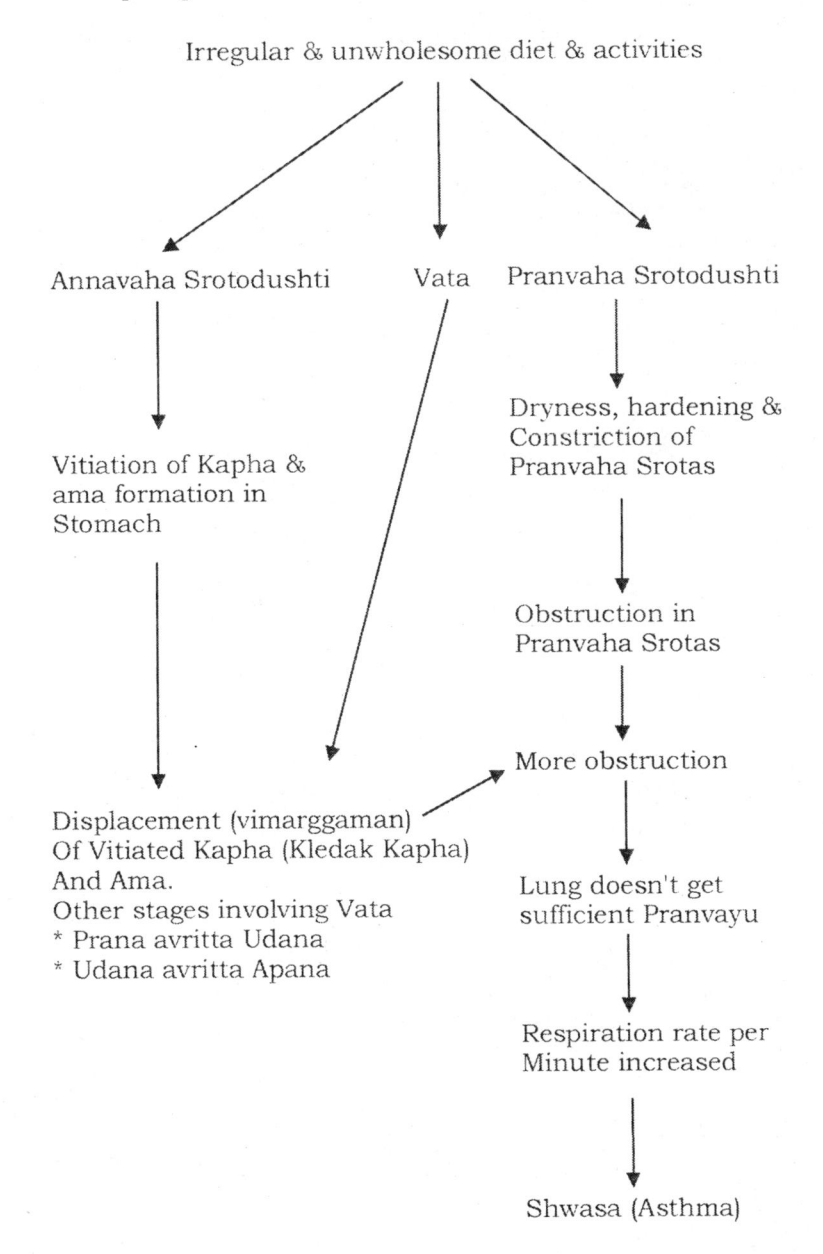

Irregular & unwholesome diet & activities

↙ ↓ ↘

Annavaha Srotodushti   Vata   Pranvaha Srotodushti

↓ ↓

Vitiation of Kapha & ama formation in Stomach

Dryness, hardening & Constriction of Pranvaha Srotas

↓

Obstruction in Pranvaha Srotas

↓

More obstruction

↓

Displacement (vimarggaman) Of Vitiated Kapha (Kledak Kapha) And Ama.
Other stages involving Vata
* Prana avritta Udana
* Udana avritta Apana

Lung doesn't get sufficient Pranvayu

↓

Respiration rate per Minute increased

↓

Shwasa (Asthma)

Etiopathogenesis of bronchial asthma

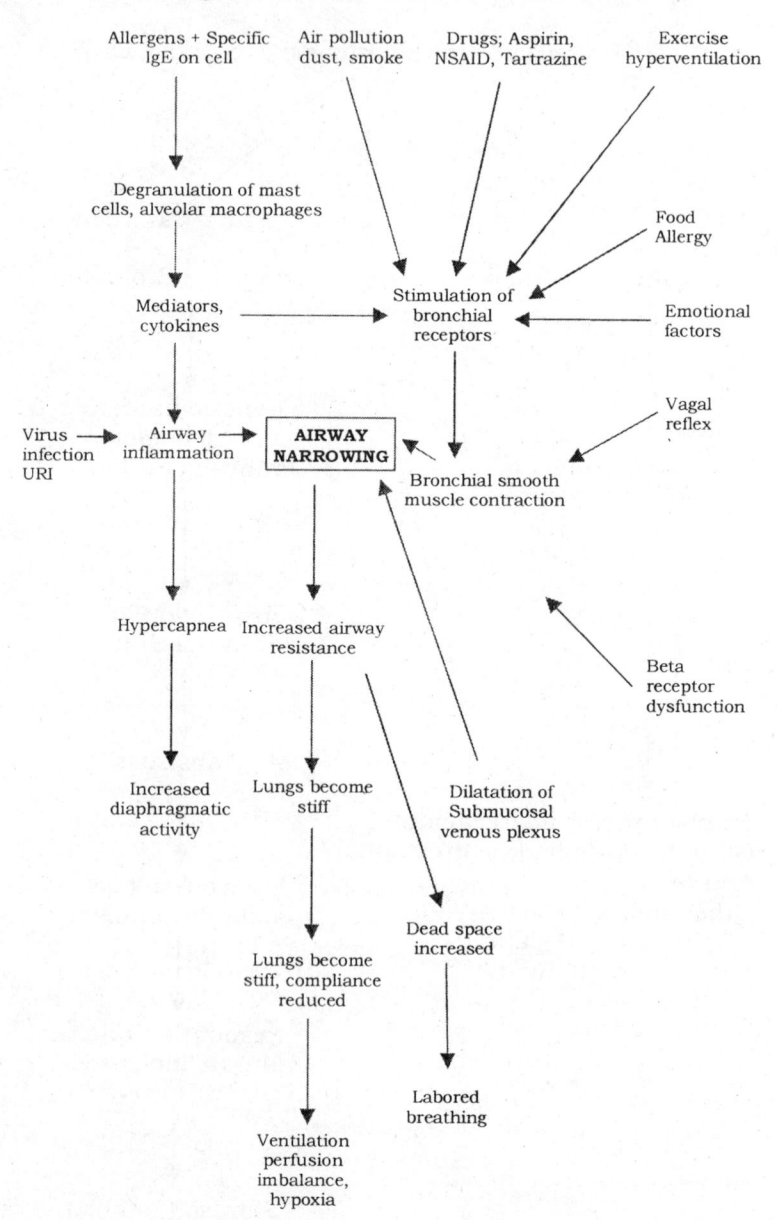

Allergens + Specific IgE on cell
↓
Degranulation of mast cells, alveolar macrophages
↓
Mediators, cytokines → Stimulation of bronchial receptors

Air pollution dust, smoke → Stimulation of bronchial receptors
Drugs; Aspirin, NSAID, Tartrazine → Stimulation of bronchial receptors
Exercise hyperventilation → Stimulation of bronchial receptors
Food Allergy → Stimulation of bronchial receptors
Emotional factors → Stimulation of bronchial receptors
Vagal reflex → Bronchial smooth muscle contraction

Stimulation of bronchial receptors → Bronchial smooth muscle contraction → **AIRWAY NARROWING**

Virus infection URI → Airway inflammation → **AIRWAY NARROWING**

Beta receptor dysfunction → **AIRWAY NARROWING**

AIRWAY NARROWING
↓
Hypercapnea | Increased airway resistance | Dilatation of Submucosal venous plexus
↓
Increased diaphragmatic activity | Lungs become stiff | Dead space increased
↓
Lungs become stiff, compliance reduced | Labored breathing
↓
Ventilation perfusion imbalance, hypoxia

SIGNS AND SYMPTOMS OF ASTHMA

1. **Maha shwasa :** The patient, when breathing, feels pain and discomfort, is not satisfied with deep breathing; there is loss of consciousness, eyes move from side to side, difficulty in closing the mouth, obstructed passage of urine and stool, inability to speak. The breathing may be heard from a distance. The patient becomes exceedingly emaciated and loses consciousness repeatedly. The mouth becomes tasteless, stool and urine become suppressed, speech becomes feeble and the mind also becomes enfeebled. This is a dangerous situation.

2. **Urdhva shwasa :** The patient can exhale, but cannot inhale properly; so, there is lack of supply of oxygen to the brain and heart. The patient looks upwards, rolls the eyes. The patient's mouth and the ducts being obstructed by phlegm, the wind, becoming excited cause considerable pain. There is great pain in the chest and head; lack of interest in life and routine activity. If neglected, he may die.

3. **Chinna shwasa :** In this type, respiration suddenly stops for a while. The patient is obliged to exert himself strongly for taking his breath, and in which the breath is inhaled slowly and in gradual puffs. A sensation in the cardiac region being torn as under is felt. Constant sweat, restless eyes, tears; emaciation and paleness of the body, redness of one of the eyes, anxiety, dryness of the mouth and delirium manifest themselves. He also suffers from Tympanitis (distension of abdomen due to accumulation of gases – *anaha*), burning sensation in the region of urinary bladder.

4. **Tamaka Shwasa :** When Vata, instead of going down, goes up, it makes the head and the neck stiff.

Kapha is aggravated, resulting in rhinitis, beginning like an attack of cold. Thereafter respiration gets obstructed and a kind of "ghar ghar" sound results. The patient gets excruciating pain in the head and chest; he often becomes unconscious. There is dry cough; when phlegm is thrown out, the patient feels relief. The throat is sore and the patient is incapable of sleeping. He cannot sleep on his back and does so in a bent position because when he makes efforts to sleep while lying on the bed, the sides of chest becomes stiff because of their affliction by aggravated vata and he gets relief in the sitting posture. There is a desire for taking hot things (fermentation, drinks). The condition gets aggravated with cold wind, blowing from the seaside. Early morning, the patient expectorates profusely, when the disease reaches the chronic stage.

Sometimes Tamaka shwasa has Pitta involvement, which is associated with fever, and fainting is called as *"Pratamak shwasa"*. It is caused by upward movement of the wind in the stomach (*udavarta*), exposure to dust, indigestion, drenching of the body, old age and respiratory obstruction.

Santamak shwasa increases by darkness and mental tension. It gets relieved by cold therapies and patient feels as if he is submerged in darkness.

In acute stage there is involvement of marmas the vital points – Shirah, Hridaya and Basti.

5. **Kshudra shwasa :** This benign type of asthma is caused by excessive intake of innutritious food and by suppression of natural urges by the consequence of the same the wind in the stomach, becoming excited, moves upwards and generates the kind of asthma known as *Kshudra* this is neither painful nor fatal. It does not obstruct the normal

passage of food and drinks; it does not cause any serious type of pain in the sense organs. It is a very minor type of painful condition.

PROGNOSIS OF ASTHMA

Mahaswasa, Urdhva Shwasa and Chinna Shwasa are incurable, as, they are the terminal complication in patients suffering from various other disorders. If Tamaka shwasa is of recent origin, and the patient has a good resistance and psychosomatic strength, it is curable. Otherwise this condition is also incurable. Only acute symptoms can be relived, not the chronic disease. Kshudra shwasa is easily curable.

Here incurable means – patient is rarely fully cured.

Symptomatically, asthma is easy to cure. In patient suffering from dysentery, heart diseases and tuberculosis, asthma is not easy to cure. If the patient of asthma and bronchitis is also suffering from hiccough, fever and vomiting, it is not easy to cure.

HOME RULES FOR ASTHMA FAMILIES

1. No smoking indoors; if you are addicted to it and can afford an adult smoking room it should be closed at all times. The asthmatic should never go into it. Stale tobacco smoke and odour are often worse than the fresh smoke.

2. Keep asthmatic children out of the kitchen when cooking causes smoke or strong odours (non-specific irritants).

3. Serve the rest of the family the same diet prescribed for the asthmatic. Separate meals separate him from the family group emotionally.

4. Be sure the asthmatic knows what he can and cannot eat. Then, as long as he sticks to it faithfully, don't discuss his diet at the table or anywhere else when he is around.

5. Don't let him eat away from home unless he can get enough of his proper foods and none of those he is allergic to.
6. Encourage him to do everything he can for himself and with his friends. Try to interest him and his friends in things that don't require too much exercise.
7. Don't talk about asthma unless what you say is interesting or helpful.
8. Don't let him get the idea that he is different or inferior.
9. Don't be overprotective, overly sympathetic, or express pity by what you say or what you do. The asthmatic child may turn out to be outstanding member of the family.
10. See to it that his dinner should be always light and must not include any greasy items with too much oil etc., and also should not be cold in potency.

WRONG PRACTICES IN DAY-TO-DAY LIFE

Intake of improper food and drinks with drugs and an irregular regimen are the main causes for diseases of body and mind. To prevent and cure such diseases, one should give up bad habits of food and conduct. In a bid to get prompt relief from disease, we take recourse of analgesics, antibiotics, steroids etc. It is often seen that a man suffering from headache due to a sleepless night at work or in a club, doesn't rest to the body and mind by sleeping for a longer time, but prefers to take a pain killer to keep himself fit. Prolonged use of these chemicals affects the vital organs – heart, brain, kidney, liver and lungs. Excessive use of steroids and sleep-inducing drugs causes extensive damage to the respiratory tract.

5

PREVENTIVE MEASURES FOR ASTHMA

The ultimate aim of Ayurveda is to prevent diseases, to achieve a normal healthy life and also to prevent asthma. A proper diet, a rational behaviour and observance of a proper regimen are advised. Therefore, Ayurveda is mainly concerned with the ways in which a life may be made good or bad, happy or unhappy. There is an ancient saying: "Prevention is better than cure", meaning that diseases can be prevent through preventive measures. In heart disease and in all the other disease like asthma, this saying has great significance. To achieve this, Ayurveda has prescribed codes of living regimen, behaviour, diet etc. For example, if a pregnant lady obeys the rules and regulations of Ayurveda during pregnancy, she can prevent congenital diseases or abnormalities of foetus and several respiratory diseases.

If asthma affects a person, it takes a lot of time to recover. He takes costly medicines and finally he may have to undergo surgical treatment, which is very risky. Recovery is possible only if these steps are taken.

Even after recovery he is likely to lose his ability to perform physical and mental work. He becomes a liability to his family. So it is good to prevent rather than cure diseases of the lungs. In preventive treatment, the way of living has to be taken care of; worry and tension need to be avoided. Excess of tea, coffee and alcohol should be avoided. One should use vegetable and fruits in large quantities. Exercise is an essential requirement for maintaining good health. Yoga is an ideal practice. Constipation should be avoided. Herbal products should be preferred over other types of preparations.

AVOIDANCE OF CAUSATIVE FACTORS OF ASTHMA

For prevention of asthma, the first line of preventive treatment is to "avoid the causes of asthma". As discussed earlier, all factors responsible for vitiation of Vata and Kapha are involved. These include excessive exercise, fasting, intake of cold water and drinks, use of dry and dirty food, suppression of natural urges, inhalation of dust and smoke, intake of heavy and oily food, use of curds and banana.

AVOIDANCE OF OVER-EATING

Instead of a heavy meal, the patient should take very light meals. Asthma is essentially a disease of over-nourishment, i.e. intake of food in excess to one's ability to digest and metabolise. Therefore, patients of asthma should generally observe periodic fasts. Asthma patients should, as a rule, take a very light meal at night or they can even avoid taking any food at all. At night when the body is at rest, the digestion and metabolism becomes very low. The patient should use some other digestive stimulants, such as rock salt, black pepper, ginger and long pepper.

AVOIDANCE OF COLD DRINKS AND SOUR JUICES

A patient of asthma should strictly avoid cold drinks, ice cream and fruit juices, particularly the juice of citrus fruits. For a healthy person, cold drinks, ice cream and fruit juice are refreshing and nourishing. But for asthmatic, these things cause a lot of damage because of their properties to cause inflammation and constriction in the bronchial tubes. These things also promote *ama* formation. Cold drinks, ice cream etc., because of their cold and oily properties vitiate Vata and Kapha (Both doshas are the chief causes of asthma).

AVOIDANCE OF TOBACCO

Tobacco, in any form, is harmful and may lead to high blood pressure or asthmatic bronchitis. Nicotine causes roughness and dryness in the body and aggravation of both Vata and Kapha. The urge to smoke indicates mental strain. One should develop the willpower to resist such rages and temptations. Smoking causes irritation in the bronchial mucosa leading to chronic bronchitis and asthmatic attacks. Some patients are allergic to tobacco fumes.

ADVERSE EFFECTS OF TEA AND COFFEE

Caffeine is present in tea and coffee. It causes hardening of the vessels, resulting in sleeplessness, anxiety and tension, thus leading to asthmatic attacks. Serving tea or coffee, has become a part of our social life today. Businessmen and administrators, take several cups of these beverages during the day and often, even at night. Excessive intake of tea and coffee should be avoided for maintaining the health of the body and the respiratory system, whereas this can be substituted with herbal tea and coffee. Ayurveda India has formulated a beverage with coffee like flavour, which can be used in any amount.

PREVENTION OF CONSTIPATION

As mentioned earlier, the places of origin of asthma are the stomach and the intestines. Constipation is an important cause for the aggravation of Vata. Those who are habitually constipated generally suffer from asthma, or patient of asthma generally suffer from constipation. The toilet habits of most of them are irregular. If the colon is blocked, the stomach and intestines do not function properly and the patient continues to suffer from asthma. Instead of taking a laxative or purgative to overcome constipation, the asthmatic patients take medicines or take specific food, which impair bowel movements. Practitioners of modern medicine find it difficult to cure patient of asthma because of the lack of holistic approach, their efforts being directed mainly towards suppression of symptoms. If an asthma patient takes a mild laxative daily, he does not require any medicine and is likely to get permanent cure if other conditions are satisfied.

Patients having chronic constipation should take water stored overnight in a copper vessel early in the morning specially the Kapha constitution people having sluggish movement of intestine (Here a vaidya must guide about the difference in the sluggish movement and dryness of the intestine which is a Vata symptom).

The best laxative for asthma patients is haritaki (*Terminalis chebula*). One teaspoonful of haritaki powder should be mixed with 1/4 teaspoonful of powdered rock salt and given to the patient at bedtime with luke warm water. Here we advise to interrupt this prescription in between as Charaka advises not to take any salt continuously for 1 month.

AVOIDANCE OF SUPPRESSION ON NATURAL URGES

Suppression of natural urges causes aggravation of Vata, which lead to asthma and lung diseases. As described earlier, there are 13 types of natural urges. Suppression of an urge to urinate and to defecate generally impairs the functioning of the kidney and the heart. It is a normal phenomenon for the body to throw out undesirable waste products. To follow the body desires timely is good for health.

ANXIETY, DESIRE, TENSION AND ASTHMA

Asthma and lung disease are closely related to mental activities. All forms of mental strain – anxiety, worry, fear and emotional stress, affect both digestion and metabolism. Disturbance in digestion leads to ama formation in the body, which is the chief cause of many diseases including asthma.

There is a common notion, that the mind is entirely different from the body. This is not correct. Almost all patient of asthma, including young patients, suffer from mental strain and emotional stress. This fact is generally ignored by the modern society. The exact cause of stress and strain should be located and removed, failing which the patient will live with asthmatic attacks. Only periodic suppression of the symptoms can be achieved by taking anti-spasmodics. As per a well-known saying, we should avoid hurry, worry and curry. It is good to be smart and active but it is bad to lead about them. If at times you fail to achieve your objectives do not indulge in excessive worry. It is not possible in this world to always achieve the objectives despite hard and sincere efforts. We have time for parties, gossips, films and other cheap modes of entertainment, but we have no time for complete relaxation of the body and mind. To be in a hurry while eating food, running to the place of work immediately after eating food, discussing family problems at the dining table and attending telephone calls and watching T.V. during meals have become a part of our life. According to Ayurveda, food should be taken in an absolutely peaceful environment, without any mental tension. The food which is consumed in a hurry may cause dyspepsia, indigestion and other diseases including liver and lung diseases. Ayurvedic philosophy is further supported in the Bhagvad Gita when Lord Krishna tells Arjuna.

"If a person follows a planned diet and daily regimen it will help to maintain health and prevent diseases."

BENEFICIAL FRUITS, VEGETABLES AND BEVERAGES

Vegetarian food being easy to digest is good for asthmatic patients. In Ayurveda, non-vegetarian food is considered to be good for certain categories of people. But they are 'tamasika' in nature. They are not good for mental health and are harmful for the heart and lungs.

Now a days, more and more vegetables and fruits are being produced in cold countries. Vegetable and fruits from one part of world can reach the other parts. But the habits are hard to change. Those who are taking non-vegetarian food continue their food habits because of false impressions created about the high nourishing value of meat, eggs, chicken etc. Whereby such food are becoming popular even in tropical countries. Scientific researches show the ill effects of non-vegetarian food but have not had adequate impact on the mind of the people.

Vegetables and fruits harmful for asthmatic patients: Ripe bananas, oranges, lemon, sour fruit juice, sour fruits, pickles, potatoes, arvi, colocasia, legumes of different types; sea fish and eggs should be avoided. Constipating vegetables should also be avoided.

Vegetables and fruits beneficial for asthmatic patients: Spinach, bitter gourd, pumpkin, green banana and papaya, grapes, raisins, garlic and ginger are good for asthma patients.

Dry ginger powder, asafoetida, cumin seeds, turmeric, long pepper, black pepper, cinnamon, cardamom and cloves are also beneficial.

FOOD AND RULES FOR EATING IN ASTHMA

To prevent lung diseases and asthma, one should avoid such ingredients in food and drinks, which cause aggravation of Vata and Kapha. Dry, rough, bitter, pungent and astringent foods aggravate Vata, whereas innutritious and heavy foods aggravate Kapha. Asthma is a disease for over-nourishment. Instead of a heavy meal, the patient should take very light meals, especially at night. He should avoid rice and should take wheat instead. However, taking refined wheat flour is not advisable, because it is constipating. Asthmatic patients should take whole-meal bread, maize and bajra (millets). Cow's milk should be preferred to buffalo milk. Goat's milk is particularly beneficial for asthmatics. It is good to add half a teaspoon of powdered long pepper or ginger to milk, tea or coffee before boiling. Alcoholic drinks can be used in moderation, though ice should be aoivded and drinks should be taken in a highly diluted state. (Exposure to cold wind, rain, dust and smoke should be avoided.)

Rules for eating food

1. Food should be warm.
2. Food should be taken in proper quantities.
3. Food should be taken after digestion of the previous meal.
4. Food should be taken at a proper place.
5. Food should be taken with concentration of mind.
6. Food should be taken neither in a hurry nor very slowly.
7. Food should be taken with self-confidence.
8. The type of and quality of food should be taken according to time, season, age and climate.

One should take sufficient quantity of water in a day for the proper functioning of the kidneys and lungs. Drinking water before meals reduces obesity, when taken during meals, it promotes strength. Drinking water after meals causes obesity. A light breakfast and two meals a day keep the body healthy. Where taking a solids, one-fourth should be filled with liquid and the remaining one-fourth kept empty for proper digestion of food. Physical exercises just after meals should be avoided because these aggravate Vata. A little rest after meals promotes longevity. Sitting for a long time just after meals make the abdomen bulge out.

Diet

Diet plays a vital role in Ayurveda treatment. By controlling and regulating the diet and also by taking appropriate nutritious diet, 50% of the disease can be taken care of. Therefore, diet is planned to suit the above three stages of treatment.

Eliminative diet

Fasting (langhan) is extensively used to induce a physiological rest while at the same time allowing the organs to begin its inner cleansing process. Although there is loss of weight during the fast, it is not its primary function. Fast is a health promoting treatment, which stimulates body's inherent power to fight disease and promote health as it burns toxins (Ama), which plays a major role in pathology of Asthma.

The patient is generally kept on fast for three or more days depending upon his general condition and constitution. During this period, he is encouraged to drink 8-10 glasses of water a day. Water helps to flush the system and eliminate large quantity of toxins and mucus. Water also saturates the dried up mucus in the system so that it is expelled more easily.

Soothing diet

In the second stage, when the patient recovers from the acute attack, he is prescribed nourishing food and non-mucus producing diet, consisting of seasonal fruits twice a day. Milk and milk products are totally avoided during the eliminative and soothing stages and also constructive stage.

Constructive diet

When the asthmatic condition is completely relieved, the patient is prescribed normal constructive food and fruits. The diet may consist of porridge, idli (a traditional South Indian dish made of steamed rice), moong dal, Brown bread with mild unsalted white butter, raisins etc.

HARMFUL EFFECTS OF CURD (YOGHURT) ON ASTHMATICS

Ayurveda prohibits the use of curd or yoghurt at night even by healthy persons. Ayurveda, categorizes curd/yoghurt as Abhisyandi that is, it obstructs the channels of circulation. At night, the process of circulation becomes very slow because of general inactivity. Curd if consumed, may further slow down the process of the body. It is considered a heavy food. In the patients of asthma, intake of curd may further slow down the circulation, which can further enhance inflammation, spasms, or constriction in the bronchial tubes.

CONTROL OF WEIGHT

Being overweight is harmful, for the body, particularly in the case of asthmatics. In most cases, asthma arises from obesity, a sedentary life style, intake of an improper diet of Vata and Kapha, food which is rich in fat, inadequate physical exercise and mental tension. Obese people are more prone to asthma. One should avoid excessive fatty and starchy foods. Dietary articles fried in oil and ghee is very harmful if consumed in excess. Morning walk and walking after dinner is beneficial.

AVOIDANCE OF EXCESSIVE USE OF DRUGS

Now a day, many young people indulge in taking opium, heroin, LSD, Dexedrine and various other intoxicating drugs. Due to a fast life and sleep-lessness, they are using mood elevators and antidepressants. In Ayurveda, opium and its by-products are used as medicine in small doses after their purification with milk, honey, ghee and lemon juice. If the patient is of a strong physical and mental constitution with Kapha dominant asthma, he should be treated with Shodhana therapy i.e. purifying measures for the body, which includes oleation, steaming, vomiting, purgation and smoking along with Kapha alleviating and anti-asthmatic herbal drugs. The type of treatment is called Aptarpana therapy. This purification rids them of their adverse effects. But their misuse of intoxication is harmful for the body and lungs, which should be strictly avoided. Excessive dependence on drugs is harmful for both the body and the mind. It is reported that in western countries, 80% of the people are taking a pill or a tablet daily for getting relief from tension, headaches, etc. This is a dangerous trend. Analgesics, steroids and antibiotics should be taken only when it is absolutely essential. Instead of taking analgesic and hypnotic drugs, one should give rest to the mind and body by meditation and massage.

USE OF PREVENTIVE DRUGS

To keep the three doshas (Vata, Pitta and Kapha) in a state of equilibrium and to protect the body against the onset of asthma, it is necessary to use some preventive drugs regularly.

- One such herbal drug for this is the plant 'Haritaki' (*Terminalis chebula*). The method for using this herb in different seasons is described in next section. Regular use of Haritaki is beneficial for any normal healthy person in general and for asthmatics in particular.
- Turmeric is another drug, which is widely used for the prevention for allergy, rhinitis and asthma. Asthma generally starts with or is associated with rhinitis or inflammation and congestion of the mucous membranes of the nose. The patient gets a few bouts of sneezing, a runny-nose and watery eyes. The infection spreads to the throat and then to the bronchial tubes, leading to asthma. Turmeric has both a preventive and a curative action against this disease. As a preventive treatment, a person should take 1 teaspoon of turmeric powder mixed with 2 teaspoons of honey twice a day on an empty stomach. He can also take 1 teaspoonful of turmeric powder mixed with a cup of warm milk, twice a day. By taking turmeric in this manner prior to the onset of a nasal problem, asthmatic attacks can be prevented.
- *Long pepper* traditionally known in Sanskrit as Pippali has been used in Ayurveda and Unani medicine in the prevention and treatment of bronchial asthma.
- *Adathoda vasica* known in Ayurveda by its Sanskrit name Vasaka has been traditionally included in preparations for the relief of cough, asthma and bronchitis. This drug is useful in clearing the airways by decreasing the mucus secretion and opening the air passages.
- *Tylophora indica* (syn: *T. asthmatica*) Sanskrit – Anthrapachaka/Anantmool. The therapeutic property of this herb is well documented in the treatment of bronchial asthma.

- *Boswellia serrata.* Sanskrit - Salai guggul. Boswellic acids derived from sap of the Boswellia tree are known to block the leukotriene biosynthesis by inhibiting enzyme lipoxygenase. This can be a drug of choice as an analgesic for the Asthmatic patients having Arthritis or some other painful musculo-skeletal disorder.
- *Coleus forskohlii* contains the diterpene derivative, forskohlin, which may activate cyclic AMP. Forskohlin has been successfully used in alleviation of experimentally induced asthma in human volunteers.

The following components are normally included in the Ayurvedic approach to the management of asthma:

Essential components:
- Long term administration of pulmonary tonics to strengthen the lungs like Chywanprash/Albiz malt.
- Administration of relaxing expectorants to prevent the building up of sputum like Banapsha (Viola odorata)
- Anti-spasmodic preparations to help mitigate the effect of the bronchospasm on the pulmonary muscles like Vasa(Adhatoda vasica), Tulsi (Ocimum sanctum), Bharangi (Clerodendrum serratum).

Ancillary components:
- Demulcents could be used to soothe irritation of mucous surfaces e.g. Yashtimadhu (Glycrrhiza glabra).
- Anti-microbial compounds would prevent secondary infections e.g Haridra,Tulsi.
- Anti-catarrhals would prevent the over pro-duction of sputum in lungs or sinuses e.g. Trikatu/Vyosh(a combination consisting equal parts of Sunthi, Maricha, Pippali).

- Nervine support herbs are needed to enable adaptation to stress. Excessive stress or nervous debility may aggravate the symptoms of asthma e.g. Jatamansi (Nordostychus jatamansi), Vacha (Acorus calamus).

  Herbal formulations used in the management of asthma are prepared by combining herbs, which provide the above characteristics.

GENERAL TIPS FOR THE PREVENTION OF ASTHMA

Asthmatic person

- Should avoid the factors, places, business, that cause asthma.
- Should avoid moist places.
- Must go for daily morning, evening walk and do yoga exercises like surya namaskar and pranayam.
- Must go to sleep in time at night.
- Should avoid constipation.
- Should avoid mental tension.
- Must brush teeth every morning and after meals and have good hygienic life.
- Must avoid tobacco, wine and smoking habits.
- Should avoid dust, fur clothes & fur animals.
- Must avoid overeating and take light dinner one hour before going to bed.
- Should not overload house with furniture and carpets.
- Should keep rooms ventilated and use exhaust fan in the kitchen.
- Should avoid air conditioners, cooler and direct air of fan.

- Must avoid perfumes, aggarbatti, mosquito repellents that aggravate attack.
- Must not over exercise, over do sex, over do work, eat 'ruksha aahar', smoke, take excess emesis and laxative and suppress toilet urge.
- Must drink boiled water in excess.
- Must avoid those medicines which aggravate asthmatic symptoms e.g. Asprin, Ibuprofen etc.

If asthmatic patient is a lactating mother, she must continue breast-feeding. It will strengthen the defense system of the child.

Parent of asthmatic students must inform the school-teacher to keep their ward out of the aggravating activities.

REGULATION OF DAILY AND SEASONAL ROUTINES

Instruction regarding the observance and regulation of ideal daily and seasonal routines consisted of some simple but effective rules of living, especially for the patients of *Tamaka Shvasa*.

Ideal daily routines

Morning

- Wake up with the sun (from 5.30 am. to 6.30 am)
- Evacuate bowel and bladder.
- Clean teeth.
- Gargle with lukewarm salt water.
- Clean tongue with tongue scraper.
- Take walk or light exercise of neuro-muscular integration.
- Practise deep breathing exercise.

- Give yourself a warm oil massage.
- Take bath (with warm water during cold weather).
- Take a light breakfast.
- Work or study.

Noon
- Take the main meal of the day.
- Take rest (not sleep) for 15 or more minutes.

Afternoon
- Work or study

Evening
- Gargle with lukewarm salt water.
- Take a light supper, the earlier the better but not latter than 7.30 p.m.
- Take a brief walk for 15 minutes.
- Practice deep breathing exercise
- Enjoy the relaxing activities, music, read-ing, chatting etc.
- Go to sleep before 10.00 p.m. (in a cozy room in winter).

6

ROLE OF YOGA IN ASTHMA

People working in offices and shops often lead a sedentary life. After work, they have very little energy left for walking, exercise or for doing any physical work. This affects digestion. Running or walking in a hurry, after taking food is harmful. But after 15 minutes rest, a person can walk.

One should practice yoga and meditation regularly if one wants to keep their body and mind in a good shapes. Apart from spiritual peace, meditation always helps in keeping the body physically healthy. Many rules are prescribed in Yoga. Yogis for asthmatic patients describe many physical postures or asanas and breathing exercises or pranayama. Before undertaking these practices some cleansing measures should be taken. These measures are called Shat karmas. They are:

1. Dhauti
2. Basti
3. Neti
4. Trataka
5. Nauli
6. Kapalabhati

Including Kunjala and Sankhpraksalana.

Each individual has specific requirements. Kunjala should be practised regularly and is very beneficial for the lungs. It involves taking saline water and vomiting it out.

Hatha yoga consists of eight different practices.

1. Yama : Practice for controlling mental aberrations.
2. Niyama : Religious performances and disciplined life habits.
3. Asana : Practice of different physical postures.
4. Pranayama : Breath control.
5. Pratyahara : Withdrawal of senses from indulging in their objectives.
6. Dharana : Concentration.
7. Dhyana : Meditation.
8. Samadhi : Deep meditation in a state of trance.

YOGIC THERAPY FOR ASTHMA

The asthma patients are exposed to the entire system of yoga therapy. Yoga therapy does not only constitute the physical aspect, but also the psychological and rejuvenative aspect as well. This can be divided into 3 distinct yet inter-related activities namely.

I. The Yoga Kriyas

These constitute Kunjal and Neti, the eliminative techniques (cleansing).

- **Effect of Neti on Asthma :** Jal neti and sutra neti (thread) are the two types. Its regular practice activates the nasal mucosa and makes them resistant to the effect of climatic changes, particularly humid climate.
- **Effect of Kunjal on Asthma :** The Kunjal (vomiting) relaxes the bronchial wall and open it to let the secretion out. In Asthma, thin bronchial walls go into spasm as mucus blocks the out-ward passage. In these processes,

excessive bile and phlegm and other impurities of the stomach and oesophagus are cleaned and sputum from the chest and trachea is removed.

Kunjal Kriya is one of the most effective yogic techniques. It is dramatic and instantaneous in its action. It can give immediate relief from asthma and from acidity, indigestion, headache, anxiety, neurosis, depression and psycho somatic problems.

Direct Effects

1. At the **physical level**, Kunjal can aid the maintenance of good health as well as help in the cure of the acidity and gas in the stomach, biliousness, nausea, food poisoning and auto poisoning, indigestion, inflamed oesophageal mucosa, coughs, asthma, bronchitis and respiratory ailments, headache and diseases of the nervous system.

2. At the **mental level**, Kunjal can help with many types of mental diseases and problems, acting as a kind of shock therapy to recharge the brain and mind. It especially helps in depression, lethargy, tensions, anxiety, neurosis and phobia.

3. At the **pranic level**, Kunjal gives the whole body a flushing, untying knots and unblocking nadis, so that the whole body feels revived and alive.

Benefits : Kunjal kriya tones up and helps to rebalance the nervous system, thus helping to rejuvenate the whole body. The energy released by the pranic flash helps tone up the circulatory system, the respiratory system, the urogenital system and the musculo-skeletal system.

When we do kunjal, we stimulate the sensory channel of our nervous system, which sends a signal to the brain. This in turn sends a signal down the motor system to make the body vomit: the diaphragm, stomach and glottis contract, causing the water to move in the reverse direction.

There are three process of the body, which totally paralyse the brain and mind for one moment, leaving you in a self-ness reminiscent state of meditation. These are orgasm, sneezing and vomiting. If you think about it and reflect upon your own experience, you will remember that at the moment of experiencing one of these three states, you felt a wave of energy rush through your body and mind which momentarily stopped all thought and action.

When the brain feels this rush of energy it is in a state of extreme stimulation. Many of its circuits are temporarily cut, leaving only the few most necessary circuits in action. This situation is analogous, but much more gentle, subtle and effective than ECT. The brain then pours out this energy, cleans and purifies by stimulating the cell of the waste-disposal system, and then travel on to the organs of the body. As a result there is a direct increase in body efficiency.

When we do Kunjal Kriya, the action of energy flush moves from the stomach on the Physical level, and *Manipura Chakra* on the Psychic level, stimulates the vagus nerve both in its sensory and motor functions. The vagus is sensory to the heart, lungs, bronchi, and digestive tract. It feeds directly into the hypothalamus of the brain via its *parasympathetic* fibres. The hypothalamus controls the whole autonomic nervous system. The vagus is responsible for the gag reflex and vomiting. The extra energy from Kunjal spills into both sympathetic and parasympathetic systems, but as the mind is prepared for vomiting, a stressful situation the sympathetic predominates.

II. Yogasana

The main asanas prescribed for asthmatic patients are Sarvangasana, Paschi-mottanasana, Janusirshasana, Bhujangasana, Gomukhasana, Ardhmatsyerndrasana, Virasana, Suptavajrasana, Padmasana, Badhpadmasana, Yoganidrasana, Shalabh-asana, Dhanurasna, Ustrasana, Urdhavadha-nurasana and Vajrasana.

These asanas are helpful in reshaping the chest and improve the body posture; strengthen the spinal cord, allow flow of pranic energy into the body. The constant and regular practice of these asana develops body resistance to ward off any external adverse condition.

The asanas that are particularly helpful to improve the breathlessness are Sarvangasana, Halasana, Paschimottanasana, Parvatasana, and Urdhvadhanur-asana.

These asanas should, however, be performed under the supervision of an expert yogi.

III. Pranayama

Pranayama is an excellent means of using the lungs to the fullest extent. By full use of the lungs and exercise, the chest cavity and the autonomic nervous system is rebalanced. The patients may practice the following variants of Pranayamas twice a day:

Anuloma Viloma, Bhastrika, Kapalabhati, Ujjayi, Suryabhedana.

THE NOSE: A PRANIC BIODETECTOR

It is established that biological sustenance is dependent upon breathing. Many yogic texts support this conclusion. Perhaps the clearest reference is in the second chapter of the Hatha Yoga Pradikpika which declares that: "As long as breathing continues, life exists; when the break departs, so too does life. Therefore regulate the breath."

The nose is very significant, for at the root of the nasal cavity is a uniquely designed prana detecting device. This is a thin, perforated bone, known in medical terminology as the cribriform plate of the ethmoid bone. Within these perforations, the minute filaments of the olfactory nerve reside. They relay information to the brain concerning the constituents of the air, when electrically charged ions contact these filaments; the brain and main nervous system automatically become energized. The charging travels to the limbic system of the brain, in which perceptions are transformed into experience. So breathing directly affects our emotional responses to life, and converse the arousal of different emotion reflected in the breath.

If one breathes through the mouth, the entire air mass and prana travel straight down to trachea without stimulating the brain and nervous system. Therefore the activation of the entire nervous system is dependent on nasal breathing.

Pranayama, is generally known as a breathing exercise. In Pranayama, the person inhales, retains and exhales breath at the rate of 1 : 2 : 4 i.e., the inhalation time should be 1; the time of retaining the breath should be 2 and that of exhalation 4. This is the commonly followed rule. There are, however, many exceptions, which one can ascertain from an expert yogi. Depending upon the strength of the patients, it can be done for one, two, four and eight minutes. During this process, the parts, which are in yogic parlance, are called Puraka, Kumbhaka and Rechaka Pranayama. The patient mind should be concentrated upon a fix point in the body, preferably near his heart, and he should try to avoid any diversion of mind. If it is practised regularly after the bowels have been cleared and on an empty stomach, two or three times a day, it gives immense mental tranquillity to the patients, enabling him to overcome stress and strain and thereby, successfully preventing asthmatic attacks.

This simple exercise teaches breathing techniques for optimal aeration. The following points merit consideration:

- In the normal condition, a person at rest inhales air 12 times and exhales the air 12 times per minute. However, most of us do not expand the chest during the process of breathing-in, adequately enough to allow the expansion of the lungs.
- We instead use the diaphragm muscle (abdominal breathing) which does not ventilate the lungs sufficiently.
- Another reason for poor aeration of lungs is that we tend to rush the cycle of breathing in and out.
- The proper ratio for exhalation should be twice the time taken for inhalation.
- The most difficult part for those in Yogic training of breath is to have a steady exhalation, without holding the breath or experiencing a choking sensation.
- Proper breathing practice would not only help alleviate the symptoms of some pulmonary conditions like asthma, but would also help to improve circulatory abnormalities like hypertension as well as provide relief from mental stress and anguish.

YOGIC BREATHING, TOTAL BREATHING

The lungs are enclosed in a cage bounded below by the diaphragm and at the sides by the chest wall. Breathing works by making the cage bigger.

Essentially, there are **three groups of muscles** responsible for the act of inspiration. They are:

- Diaphragm, which is a muscular sheath separating the chest from the abdominal cavity, and is the main component. (Unfortunately, most people don't make use of it). Diaphragm is a convex dome. When it contracts it flattens and increases the space above; thus allowing air to be sucked into the lungs.

- Intercostal group of muscles, placed in between the ribs they are responsible for expansion of the chest. They cause the ribs; to move up and out, increasing the space available.
- Accessory group, essentially neck muscles above clavicle that is rarely used in normal daily breathing.

During normal relaxed breathing, your stomach will gently move up and down as you breath in and out. This is due to the fact that the diaphragm presses down on contents of your stomach during inspiration causing it to bulge out. A newborn child breathes with the abdomen. As the child gets older, breathing becomes partially intercostal (i.e. chest breathing). During adult life most of us breathe only through the chest. Abdominal breathing (maximal use of the diaphragm) is almost forgotten. So much so that when the person tries to inhale, his chest expands but the abdomen moves in, which is abnormal. It makes the breathing process less effective. Lower lobes of the lungs are perfused with greater amount of blood than the upper and middle lobes. By abdominal breathing lower lobes get properly ventilated. Unfortunately, most people do not make use of their diaphragm, and breathe with the help of their chest muscles. If all the movement comes from your chest then not only are you underutilizing the capacity of your lungs, but your breathing is also less relaxed.

It has been noted that during sleep and relaxed state the breathing automatically becomes abdominal. During anxiety state breathing becomes rapid and is fully intercostal. When the individual purposely breathes slowly and deeply through the abdomen the effect of stress on the body is reduced. This is borne out by favourable change in the brain wave pattern (alpha) during slow abdominal breathing.

To practise abdominal breathing, sit comfortably with your back straight. Always breathe through the nose which filters warm air. Place your right hand on the chest and left hand on your abdomen. This will help you to be aware of your abdominal muscles as you breathe. As you begin to inhale, your left hand on the abdomen should begin to rise, but your right hand should move very little. Now exhale as much air as you can while contracting your abdominal muscles. Once again your left hand should move in as you exhale but your right hand should move very little. This is abdominal breathing. Breathing through your abdomen will gradually become automatic if you practice it on regular basis. If you are having a hard time learning abdominal breathing, then lie on the floor in the resting position and gently place a soft weight (small book) on your abdomen. Abdominal breathing will cause the weight to rise and fall with your respirations.

Pranayama means control of the pranic energy. It is achieved through the control of respiration.

Pranayama does not mean inspiring a greater volume of air, or utilizing more oxygen, but still, certain physio-logical figures are worth mentioning.

During ordinary, quiet breathing, going on unconsciously at the rate of 14 to 18 breathes per minute, one utilizes 500 ml of air per breath. This is known as the tidal volume.

There is no exchange of gases in the trachea and the bronchi, which are tubular structures for mere passage of air. Out of the 500 ml of tidal volume air, about 150 ml of air is wasted in this dead space. After breathing in quietly (Puraka), one can still take in a lot of entire air by conscious inspiration. Similarly after quiet breathing out (Rechaka), one can still force out a lot more air. This is known respectively as inspiratory and expiratory reserve volumes (IRG & ERV).

If one takes a deep breath after forcefully emptying the chest, one can breathe in 4,000 ml of air. This is called the vital capacity (VC). Out of this, only 150 ml is lost in the dead space. This is one of the advantages of deep breathing, which is common to all types of deep breathing and not only to yogic breathing alone.

The further advantage of yogic breathing lies in the fact that it is more a vertical breathing than horizontal.

The exercises with the chest expander, or the tape measurements of expanded and unexpanded chest, indicate a preference for horizontal expansion of the chest.

However, the yogic process of performing pranayama in a fixed sitting posture, breathing through alternate nostrils or the Ujjai, Sheetali or Sheetakari way of inspiration, promote vertical breathing. By this vertical breathing all the alveoli of both the lungs open out evenly. This effect is more obvious in the apical, central and basal alveoli.

Due to the even expansions of all the alveoli, a vast expense of alveolar membrane is available for exchange of gases. This surface is about 50 square meters in extent, which is 20 times the entire body surface. The larger the surface available for the process of diffusion, the better is the process. Moreover, if some alveoli remain unopened, they get stuck. There is a collection of secretion in them, and they are prone to disease formation. This is done away with the vertical breathing.

The diaphragmatic muscle between the chest and the abdominal cavities plays a major role in the act of respiration. It has an excursion of one cm during quite breathing, but during deep vertical breathing it moves 2-3 cm. The base of the heart and lungs are attached to the upper surface of the diaphragm, while the liver, spleen, stomach and pancreas are immediately under the diaphragm. The circulation in these organs is improved and consequently their performance is stimulated. The lymphatics below the diaphragm are also thoroughly emptied.

As against these advantages of vertical breathing, the horizontal expansion of the chest has certain disadvantages. In horizontal breathing, the alveoli towards the periphery expand more than optimum, while the centrally placed alveoli do not open out properly this affords a lesser and uneven surface for diffusion of gases. The consequences of alveoli remaining closed are many.

If the peripheral alveoli open wider than preferable, they lose their elasticity. They remain in a fixed wide-open position, with very little excursion for taking in air. The chest looks big and barrel shaped, but does not move well with respiration. The interalveolar walls may be broken, damaging the capillaries, leading to diseases like emphysema or cor pulmonale.

Thus, by yogic total, vertical breathing we include 4,000 ml of air per breath. We offer an even surface of 50 sq. meters for exchange of gases. Due to even expansion of the alveoli, we not only keep lungs intact in structure and function. We keep them healthy. We can prevent diseases like emphysema and also gain relief in asthma and chronic bronchitis. The increased amplitude of the movements of the diaphragm improves the functions of stomach, liver, spleen, heart and the circulation in the lymphatics, thus improving digestion.

Pranayama thus acts directly on the various systems of the body, and affords benefits to them all.

Proper breathing depends on our eliminating tension, correcting bad habits, wrong mental and physical attitudes; the moment we get rid of these obstacles it will come into its own and bring us vitality and good health.

SCIENTIFIC YOGIC LIFESTYLE PROGRAMME HELPFUL IN REVERSING THE BRONCHIAL ASTHMA

1. Shatkarma plus other specialized yogic purificatory techniques
2. Yogasanas (Yogic postures)
   (a) Paschimottanasana (Posterior stretch)
   (b) Shavasana (Posterior stretch)
   (c) Vrikshasana (Head-stand)
3. Pranayama (Body-mind energizing breathing practices)
   (a) Surya-bhedana (Right Nostrilar Pranayama)
   (b) Lome-vilome (Alternate Nostrilar Prana-yama), Nadi Sodhna
   (c) Bhastrika (Bellow Pranayama)
   (d) Ujjayi (Hising Pranayama)
4. Mudras and Bbandhas
   (a) Maha Bandha
   (b) Uddiyana Banda (Abdominal lock)
   (c) Moola Bandha (anala lock)
5. Dhyana (Meditation)
6. Yogic dietary regimen as per prescription
7. Fasting as per requirement

7

CURATIVE TREATMENT

For the treatment of asthma in Ayurveda, the patients are considered under two broad categories:

1. If the patient is of a strong physical and mental constitution with Kapha dominant asthma, he should be treated with Shodhana therapy i.e. purifying measures for the body, which includes oleation, streaming, vomiting, purgation and smoking in this particular disease with the help of Kapha alleviating and anti-asthmatic herbal drugs. This type of treatment is called as Apatarpana therapy.

2. If the patient is not strong physically and psychologically or weak with a Vata dominant disease, he can be cured through Vata alleviating measures and it is termed as Santarpana therapy.

MANAGEMENT

During Acute condition

Follow these steps during attack :
- Shunthi powder (Dry Ginger) 1/4th teaspoon.
  Kali Mirch (Black Pepper) 6 in number.
  Kala Namak (Rock Salt) 1/4th teaspoon.
  Tulsi leaves crushed (Ocimum Sanctum Leaves) 5 in number.

Boil this mixture in 200 ml of water, when it reduces to 50 ml, filter and sip it.
- Apply warm Sesame oil mixed with a pinch of rock salt over the chest and back region.
- Keep both feet in salted hot water.
- During an actual crisis, inhaling an antispasmodic oil is the only practical herbal help, and direct sniffing from the oil bottle, or some drops put on a tissue, will be safer than a steam inhalation, as the heat of the latter will increase any inflammation of the mucous membranes and make the congestion even worse.

Hyssop : *Hyssopus officinalis*

Aniseed : *Pimpinella anisum*

Lavender : *Lavandula officinalis*

Pine : *Pinus sylvestris*

- Rosemary : *Rosemarinus officinalis*

This management will immediately normalize the increased *Vata* and *Kapha* of the patient and relieve the tightness of the chest.

During Chronic condition

As in *Tamaka Svasa, Vata* moves upward in the passage of respiration, results in the accumulation of *Kapha* in throat and head; together they produce running of nose, bubbling sound in the throat, thus increase the respiration greatly.

> "*Pratilomama Yada Vayu Srotamsi Pratipadhyate,
> Grivama Sirasca Samgraha Sleshm Anam Samudriys Ca
> Karoti Pinasama Tene Ruddho Ghurghurkam Tatha
> Ativa Tivravegama Ca Svasam Pranaprapidakam.*"
>
> *Charak Chikitsa 17/56*

Although the *Shwasa Roga* is manifested in respiratory system yet the seat of its actual occurrence is in GIT.

"Kafavatatmakavetau Pittasthana Samudbhavau."

Charak Chikitsa 17/8

Ayurveda maintains that no approach to health can be effective unless proper preventive and purificatory measures are observed simultaneously to restore the normal physiological health.

This preventive and purificatory management course includes the diet programme, regulation of daily and seasonal routines and purification therapy.

Important : During treatment of chronic asthma, the Agni has to be corrected and breathlessness cured, i.e., the site of origin and the site of manifestation has to be taken care of. During treatment proper equilibrium between Kapha and Vata has to be recorded or maintained. The treatment should always begin with the correction of Agni and Vata. If the Agni is stimulated, there is sympathetic reflex in the lungs and mucus comes out. Obstructions in the channels of circulation have to be cleared.

1. First of all, the patient should be given a massage with salted sesame oil. This helps in melting the Kapha doshas.

2. Then the sweating therapy should be applied.

   After this, some heavy food should be given to the patient and finally, *vamana* (therapeutic vomiting) should be induced.

   Dhumpan(Medicated smoking) is useful after vomiting. The patient softly inhaling the smoke of the fruit, stem and the leaves of Datura metal from a "Hooka", may alleviate the intensity of the asthmatic breathing.

   Take Cedrus deodar, Sida cordifolia, and Nordostachys jatamansi, reduce them to paste and make a hollow stick of it, dry it in the sun, leave it in the ghee and let the patient smoke like that of a Cigar.

3. *'Tamake Tu virechanam'* it means that in *Tamaka swasa*, purgation therapy is useful in patients with bronchitis. Virechana(therapeutic purgation) helps to break the pathogenesis. Bowels should be cleared even if the patient does not feel constipated. Conditions are aggravated by psychic factors. Give light food and avoid indigestion.

4. To alleviate Kapha and Vata, Trikatu the "three pungent drugs" are useful. In chronic stages, long pepper is beneficial. Simultaneously, to promote strength, honey is given, as it also acts against Kapha. Hing (asafoetida) brings Vata down.

Special Curative Medicines

- A powder prepared by mixing 3 parts haritaki with 1 part of rock salt (adding rock salt to haritaki) clears the bowels. Haritaki is hot and has a special action on the lungs and heart.

- If there is excessive phlegm, a mixture of haritaki and old jaggery (1 year old or more) in equal proportions should be given at bedtime and in the morning.

- If Kapha is aggravated, a mixture of ginger powder and jaggery in equal portion gives relief. Jaggery by itself is good for asthma (sorry to Diabetics).

  In case of bronchial asthma caused by allergy, turmeric is given in different forms. 4-5 teaspoonfuls of turmeric along with 1 teaspoonful of butter; add a little jaggery powder and give 3-5 times in case of acute attack.

- **Chyavanprash** - The main ingredient of this herbal paste is Amalaki *(Emblica officinalis)*, the richest source of natural vitamin C. A special feature of this fruit is that, its vitamin content is not lost on exposure to heat, which happens with other drugs and fruits containing Vitamin C. Chyavanprash is a very effective remedy for asthma. 5-10gms of Chyavanprash should be taken twice a day, preferably with milk.

It is a slow-acting remedy especially beneficial in chronic cases with an effective immunomodulation.

- Ginger juice with honey liquefies the phlegm.
- Inhalation of smoke released from Vasa (leaves) and Dhatura (leaves and seeds) rolled together into cigarette form or burnt in a vessel gives temporary relief.
- The intensity of an eosinophlia attack can be reduced with the use of turmeric powder.

Antiasthmatic malt-Albiz malt (paste)

We have formulated a unique combination in the form of malt, giving remarkable results. It contains a group of herbs, which are time tested and proven antiasthmatic, with immunomodulating and free radical scavenging properties.

Its main ingredients are: Sirish (Albezia lebbeck), Sariva (Hemidesmus indicus), Rasanjan (Berberies aristata), Munakka (Vitis vinifera), Saunth (Zingiber offinale), Marich (Piper nigrum), Piper (Piper longum), Dalcini (Cinnamomum zeylanicum), Ela (Elttaria cardamomum), Brahmi (Bacopa moneiri), Amaltas (Casia fistula), Pravalpishti, silver foil, pure ghee, honey etc.

It is prescribed in a dose of 10 gm, twice a day for adults and dosage can be reduced according to age in children.

It is very useful in asthma, bronchitis, laryngitis, tonsillitis, emphysema, sinusitis, exertional breathlessness, allergic sneezing, cough etc.

Bronchial Asthma and Panchkarma (Ayurveda Cleansing Therapies)

According to ancient Ayurvedic texts, there are some purifying methods for the elimination of toxins from the body. Bronchial asthma is a chronic respiratory disorder, which results due to a continuous production of ama by improper digestion and metabolism (in large intestines). Further more ama gets deposited in the minute bronchioles and fine respiratory channels and thereby causing blockage of these channels. In the true definition of Ayurveda, this condition is called blockage of Pranavahasrotas. So removing the blockage of Pranavahasrotas, i.e. respiratory channels is the prime aim while treating this disease and removal of the blockage is only possible by Ayurvedic cleansing therapies.

The Ayurvedic cleansing therapy has five procedures (Panchkarma) for getting rid of the allergens from the body resulting in a permanent and long lasting cure of this difficult but treatable disease. Panchkarma is a purifying therapy and a healing technique used in deep-rooted chronic diseases as well as in imbalance of doshas due to impact of season and to eliminate the toxins to keep the person always healthy and rejuvenated. By eliminating toxins, the vitiated doshas, whatever the cause may be, get eliminated.

Poorva karma : (Pre procedures)
1. Oleation (Snehana) – External as well as internal.
2. Sudation (Swedana) – Steam therapy by different modes using herbal medication.

Panchkarma : (Main procedures)

The following five types of procedures are included in the Panchkarma cleansing therapies.

1. Vamana — Use of emetics (to eliminate the vitiated Kapha dosha)
2. Virechana — Use of purgatives (to eliminate the vitiated Pitta dosha).
3. Anuvasana Vasti — Use of oleous medicaments by anal route as enema therapy.
4. Nirooha Vasti — Use of decoctions made of of some crude herbal extracts, by anal route as enema therapy.

   By these two vastis alternatively or planned otherwise, the vitiated vata dosha is restored to a balanced state.
5. Shirovirechana or Nasya — Use of herbal medicaments and medicated oils or ghrita through nostrils. The entire Panchkarma treatment plan is preceded by two procedures.

Method of Panchkarma : The patient suffering from Shwasa should be administered Sveda (Sudation) first, anointing the body with oil mixed with salt. By these, the solid Kapha adherent in the channels gets liquefied and comes into the alimentary tract, which makes its expulsion easy, where by the channels become soft and thus Maruta (Vata) gets its (normal) downward movement.

After sudation, the patient should be made to eat rice mess, mixed with ghee or with dahi (curd). Then, a mild emesis therapy should be given, especially for those who have cough, vomiting, catching pain in the region of the heart and diminution of voice, by using Pippali, Saindhava and honey, which is not opposed to Vata (which does not aggravate vata).

When the Kapha gets expelled from the vitiated body (channels of the lungs especially) there will be great comfort, the channels being clear, anila (vata) begins to move unhindered. Rice-mess mixed with matulunga, amlavetasa, hingu, pilu and vida should be consumed, this acts as anulomana (laxative).

Next, a purgative drug mixed with saindhava and any sour fruit followed by warm water should be administered to produce purgation.

Since shwasa is born from the obstruction of the passage of prana vayu by kapha, it is beneficial to clear the passage by administration of purifactory therapy of both the upper and lower parts of the body. By the obstruction of the passages the internal fluid becomes greatly increased (and obstruct the passages), so also anila (vata) obstructs the passages. Hence its passage should also be cleared. If by the above treatment the disease does not subside, the kapha dosha adherent deep inside should be removed out by inhalation of smoke (of drugs) after purifying the patient by emesis and purgation therapies.

Leaves of haridra, root of eranda, laksha, manasshila, devadaru, ela, and mansi are made into a paste and a cigarette prepared. It should be lubricated with ghee and smoked; or smoke of yava mixed with ghee; or smoke of madhucchista, sarjarasa and mixed with ghee; or smoke of aguru or of chandana or guggulu, of manovaha or of resin of sala, sallaki, guggulu, aguru or padmaka – each one lubricated with ghee.

Svedana (sudation therapy) is essential for those who are fit for it and even those who are unfit should be given sudation for a short duration either by pouring warm milk mixed with sugar or oil; or by utkarika and upanaha (warm poultices) especially over the chest and throat.

Decoction of Dashmula, Shathi, Raasana, Bharangi, Bilva, Riddhi, Pushkara, Amalaki, Amruta and Nagara should be consumed; after it is digested, peya (thin gruel) processed by the same drugs should be taken.

A mud pot smeared inside with ghee should be coated (inside) with the paste of Pippali, Pippalimula, Pathya, Jantughna and Chitraka. After the paste dries up; the pot is filled with Takra (buttermilk) and kept undisturbed for a month; this is carminative and cures dyspnoea and coughs. Jivanti, Musta, Surasa, Tvak, Ela, Pushkara, Aguru, Bharangi, Nagara, Karkata, Krishna, Nagakesar are made into fine powder and mixed with sugar, double its quantity; used as when desired, it cures pain in the flanks, fever and cough and relieves hiccup and dyspnoea.

Classical treatment

- Shwasa Kuthara Rasa
- Shwasa Kasa Chintamani Rasa
- Vardhaman Pippali Yoga Rasayana

Take powdered Long Pepper in increasing doses starting from 250 mg, twice a day for eight days. Then constant dose of 4 gms for 21 days should be taken.

Boil powder of Long Pepper with 250 ml milk and 250 ml water, drink it when all water is evaporated and only milk is left over.

(I) Churna

    (a) Shatayadi Churna - Ref. Bhaishajya - Ratnavali Shwas Chikitsa.

    (b) Haridradi Churna - Ref. Bhaishajya Ratnavali Shwas Chikitsa

    (c) Shringyadi Churna - Ref. Bhaishajya Ratnavali Shwas Chikitsa

    (d) Sitopaladi Churna - Ref. Bhaishajya Ratnavali Rajyakshama

    (e) Talisadi Churna - Ref. Chakradutt

(II) Lauha

Pippaladya Lauha - Ref. Bhaishajya Ratnavali- Shwasa Chikitsa

(III) Rasa Kalpa

(a) Shwas Kuthar - Ref. Bhaishajya Ratnavali - Shwas Chikitsa

(b) Shwas Kaasa Chintamani Rasa - Ref. Bhaishajya Ratnavali - Shwas Chikitsa

(c) Swarnavasant Malati - Ref. Bhaishajya Ratnavali

(IV) Asava

Kanakasava - Ref. Bhaishajya Ratnavali - Shwasa Chikitsa

(V) Ghrita

Tejovatyadya Ghrita - Ref. Bhaishajya Ratnavali - Shwasa Chikitsa

(VI) Bhasma

(a) Abhrak - Ref. Ras Raj Sunder

(b) Raupya - Ref. Rasendra Saar Sangraha

(c) Shrung Bhasma - Ref. Ras Tarangini

(d) Suvarna Bhasma - Ref. Siddhayog Sangraha

(e) Moti Bhasma - Ref. Ras Tarangini & Rasendra Saar Sangraha

(f) Tankan Bhasma - Ref. Ras Tarangini

(VII) Arishta

Draksharishtha - Ref. Bharat Bhaishajya Ratnakar

(VIII) Pishthi

Praval Pishthi - Ref. Ayurved Saar Sangraha
Moti Pishthi - Ref. Ayurved Saar Sangraha
Agastya Haritaki
Haridra Khand

Actions indicated for the processes behind this disease

Pulmonary tonics are important in long term strengthening of the lungs, but will do little in short-term relief of an attack e.g chyvanprash and Albiz malt.

Expectorant remedies ensure that there is minimum build up of sputum in the lungs. However, stimulant expectorants would potentially aggravate the breathing difficulties. Thus, only use relaxing expectorants — bharangi and haritaki.

Demulcents will be soothing and support the relaxing expectorants e.g yashtimadhu

Anti-spasmodic plants will ease the spasm response in the muscles of the lungs, e.g. somalata and vasa.

Anti-microbial support is given in case of secondary infection, e.g. haridra.

Anti-catarrhals aid the body in dealing with over-production of sputum in lungs or sinuses, e.g. Tulsi and long pepper.

Cardio-Tonic herbs will support the heart in the case of lung congestion or strain, e.g. shati and pushkarmula.

Nervine support is always appropriate as stress is a trigger or because the asthma becomes a source of stress & concern which then in turn triggers attacks, e.g. vacha.

System support

Tonic support of the systems most affected by asthma is often the key to successful treatments. Of primary importance is, of course, the respiratory system. In addition to this, consideration must also be given to the cardio-vascular, nervous, and digestive systems. The digestive system comes into play because of any dietary sensitivity, which often has an impact on the histological structure of the alimentary canal.

8

HERBAL TREATMENT

THE HERBAL APPROACH

The increased popularity of synthetic drugs in the treatment of asthma in recent years has been attributed to their clinically proven efficacy and easy patentability. However, more recently, herbal approaches have regained their popularity, with their efficacy and safety aspects being supported by controlled clinical studies. For example, an antileukotriene drug has recently been approved for the treatment of asthma. The herbal approach offers an effective alternative antileukotriene product a boswellic acid that is derived from Shallaki (Boswellia serrata).

The care for the respiratory tract should be stressed more often now a day, especially in view of a dramatic increase in the incidence of life-threatening conditions like asthma. The human respiratory tract is universally exposed to air pollution and rapidly changing atmospheric conditions, e.g. transition from the air-conditioned car or room to blazing heat of the street, pressurized conditions of the plane cabin.

Contemporary challenges to the well being of the respiratory tract, including cigarette smoke and second hand smoke, make it particularly important to reach towards the wisdom generated by thousands of years of experience, contained in Ayurveda and related medical traditions of the Orient. Some herbal alternatives employed in these traditions are proven to provide symptomatic relief and assist in the inhibition of disease development as well. These herbs, therefore, have multi-faceted roles to play in the management of asthma.

ANTI ASTHMATIC HERBS

Most of the cases of Asthma owe their origin to ignorance or negligence of simple things in day-to-day life. Once the condition appears, taking medicines becomes unavoidable. In Ayurveda, several herbal plants and their products are recommended for preventive and curative treatment of asthma. Many of these plant-derived herbs are useful in the treatment of asthma as well as several other diseases. These drugs have been used in India and neighbouring countries for thousands of years.

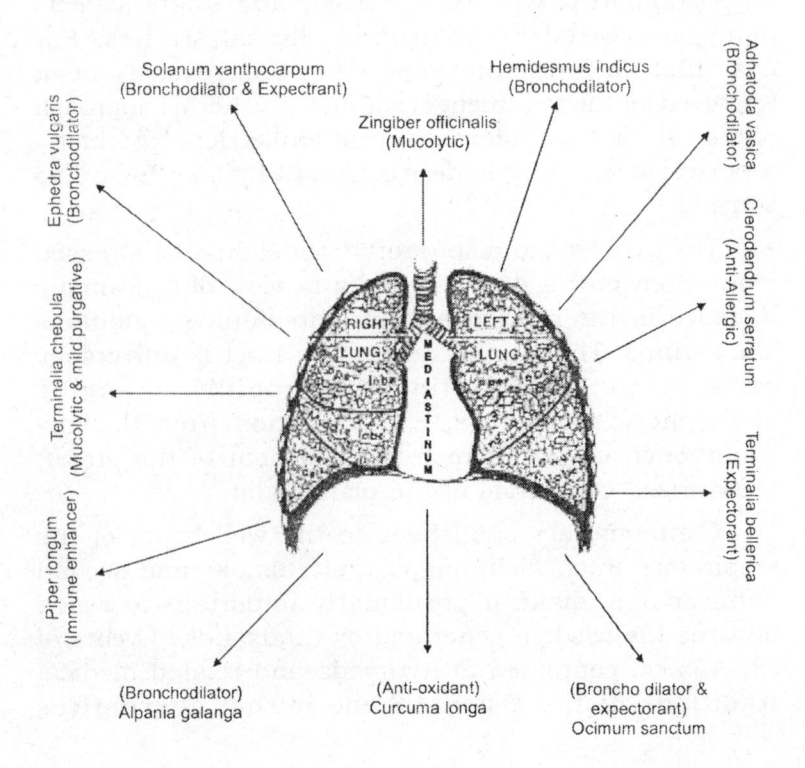

Ephedra vulgaris (Bronchodilator)
Solanum xanthocarpum (Bronchodilator & Expectrant)
Zingiber officinalis (Mucolytic)
Hemidesmus indicus (Bronchodilator)
Adhatoda vasica (Bronchodilator)
Terminalia chebula (Mucolytic & mild purgative)
Clerodendrum serratum (Anti-Allergic)
Piper longum (Immune enhancer)
Terminalia bellerica (Expectorant)
(Bronchodilator) Alpania galanga
(Anti-oxidant) Curcuma longa
(Broncho dilator & expectorant) Ocimum sanctum

There are no side effects of these drugs; rather, they have side benefits.

Ayurveda is an example of a long-standing tradition that offers a unique insight into comprehensive approach to asthma management through proper care of the respiratory tract. This includes maintaining the nourishing functions of the lungs in providing oxygen to the body.

In Ayurveda, respiratory tract functions are interrelated with those of another organ that introduces nourishment to the body, viz., the stomach. It is believed there that Kapha (which is one of the three basic dosha) is produced in the stomach and then accumulates in the lungs. Correcting imbalances in the basic doshas is critical to health and can be achieved through proper digestion and metabolism. Ayurvedic formulations used in the management of asthma, therefore, judiciously combine herbs for breathing support with antioxidant herbs such as *Curcuma longa*, herbs to support the digestive, cardiac and nerve functions, expectorant herbs as well as soothing herbs.

These herbs are natural and their uses are based upon the basic principles of Ayurveda. The herbs, besides curing asthma also act as tonics for asthma patients. Herbal treatment is relatively cheap. Several compound preparations are described in Ayurvedic texts, but in this chapter only simple forms of herbal preparations conforming to international regulations are described.

The herbs can be given to patients as well as to healthy people. In patients, these herbs cure root cause of the disease. They make the body resistant to future attacks of asthma and they do not produce any adverse effects when administered even for long periods. There is no fixed course of treatment of asthma. The administration of the drugs can be safely continued till the patient becomes absolutely free from the disease. Unlike modern medicine, no synthetic chemicals are added in these preparations.

These drugs work primarily at the sites of origin of asthma, i.e. the seat of Agni (stomach and intestines). They simultaneously correct the channels of circulation, help in removal of waste products from the body, prevent the production of these waste products and correct the site of manifestation of the disease (lungs). These plant products have anti-allergic effects and they are antispasmodic. All of them liquefy phlegm and act as

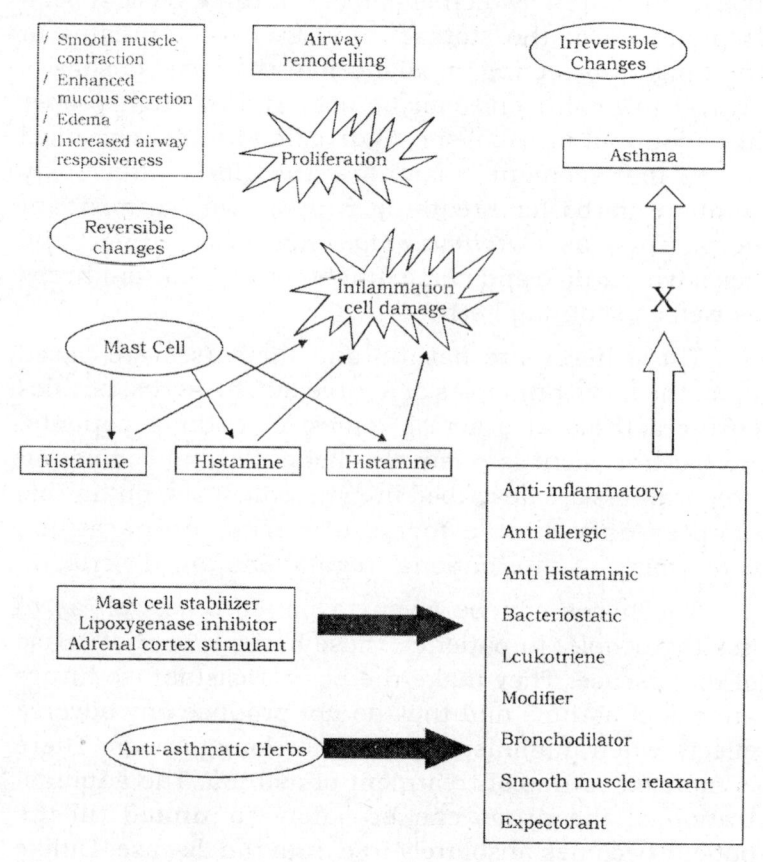

Molecular mechanism of action of Anti-asthmatic Herbs

- Smooth muscle contraction
- Enhanced mucous secretion
- Edema
- Increased airway resposiveness

Airway remodelling → Proliferation

Irreversible Changes → Asthma

Reversible changes

Inflammation cell damage

Mast Cell → Histamine, Histamine, Histamine

X

Mast cell stabilizer
Lipoxygenase inhibitor
Adrenal cortex stimulant
→
Anti-inflammatory
Anti allergic
Anti Histaminic
Bacteriostatic
Leukotriene Modifier
Bronchodilator
Smooth muscle relaxant
Expectorant

Anti-asthmatic Herbs →

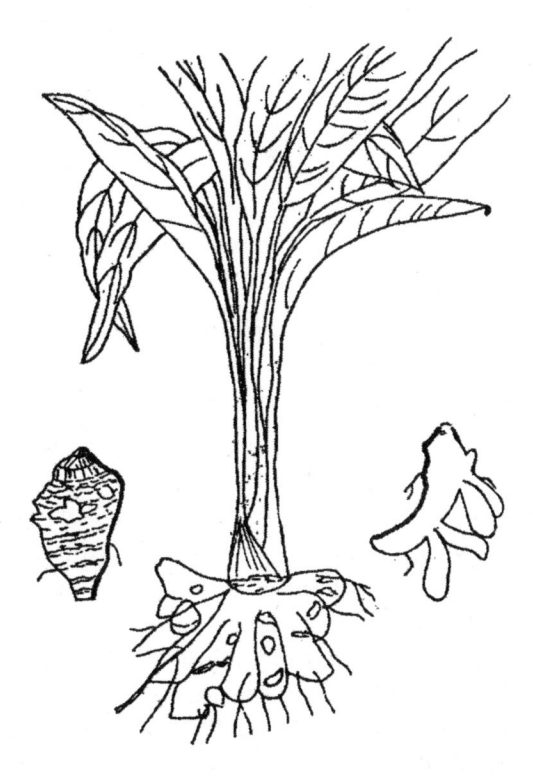

expectorants. They suppress inflammation of the bronchial tubes and promote circulation in the alveoli. In elderly patients suffering from emphysema and bronchiectasis, these plant products give immense relief.

While using these herbs, patient are advised to follow the prescribed dietary regimen and behaviour and follow the various precautions mentioned earlier.

Haridra (Curcuma Longa)

The drug has different names in different languages:

| Arabic | : | Aquid hindi |
| Enlgish | : | Turmeric |

Haridra (Curcuma longa)

French	: Curcuma, Safrandes indes
German	: Bilburir zei
Persian	: Dar-ardi
Urdu	: Haldi

It is cultivated throughout the tropical region. It is a tall herb, about 60 cm. high with large leaves. Flowers appear in the rainy season. The rhizome is used for the medicine.

ACTION ON DOSHA (BIOLOGICAL FORCES)	Pacifies Kapha, Pacifies Vata & Pacifies Pitta
GENERAL TEXTUAL INFORMATION	Anti inflammatory, Antiseptic antihelminthic.
THERAPEUTIC VALUE TEXT	Bhavprakash, Dhanvantari Nighantu, Sodhal Nighantu, Nighantu-Ratnakar, Shaligram-Nighantu.
CHAPTER	P-157.
PROPERTIES	**Rasa (Taste)** - Bitter, Pungent. **Guna (Quality)** - Light (Laghu), dry (Ruksha). **Virya (Virility)** - Hot (Ushna) potency. **Vipaka (Post assimilative effect)** - Pungent.
ACTIONS/INDICATIONS/ INSTRUCTIONS	The rhizomes are bitter thermogenic, anti-inflammatory and tonic. It is useful in ulcers, wounds, leprosy, skin diseases, pruritis, allergic conditions & discoloration of the skin.

In view of the fact that free radicals have been implicated in the pathology of asthma, the possible role of dietary antioxidants in decreasing the incidence of asthma has been explored. Deficiency of dietary Vitamin C and low levels of dietary selenium have been correlated with increased incidence of asthma in epidemiological studies. Reduced levels of glutathione peroxidase have also been observed in asthma patients.

Curcuma longa, by virtue of its antioxidant properties is an effective anti-asthmatic agent. Ayurvedic practitioners have employed it since ancient times in the treatment of respiratory disorders. The active ingredients, the curcuminoids, are potent inhibitors of inflammatory prostaglandins. The overall anti-inflammatory action of curcuminoids is also related to their well-known antioxidant properties. For example, curcumin inhibited lipid peroxidation, a phenomenon associated with antioxidant as well as anti-inflammatory activities. The well-researched antioxidant properties indicate potential use as ancillary agents in the management of asthma.

Uses : It is often used as a food supplement and is added to the curry powder. Externally, it is used in the treatment of scabies, itching, eczema, boils and abscesses. Internally, it is used for the treatment of asthma, cough, cold, fever, urticaria, jaundice, eosinophilia, throat cancer and constipation.

The rhizome of the plant is dried and ground to a powder. The paste of turmeric is mixed with an equal quantity of neem leaves and ground with water. It is applied externally and rubbed over the affected skin. Turmeric paste and powder are used internally with equal quantity of honey or sugar. In the treatment of asthma and bronchitis, it is used along with honey and ginger juice. Adding a little long pepper paste or powder fortifies its antispasmodic and expectorant properties. For bronchial asthma and chronic bronchitis associated with eosinophilia, turmeric powder is heated in cow's milk, butter or ghee. The roasted powder is used in a dose of 5 g three times a day with hot water or honey.

Dose : Turmeric powder should be given in doses of one teaspoonful (5 g) three times a day or it can be mixed with warm water or milk. Some sugar may be added.

Somlata (Ephedera Vulgaris)

The names of this herbs in different languages are:

English : Ephedra
Japanese : Maoh, Mupen
Hindi : Soma

Properties

Taste : Pungent, Bitter
Quality : Light, Sharp
Virility : Hot
Post-assimilative effect : Pungent

Somlata is a small erect shrub, a few inches in size. Its branches are dark green in colour and it is cylindrical in shape. Fruits are ovoid, red and sweet. The rhizome is large and of the size of a football. It grows in dry areas in the altitude range of 7,000-16,000 ft.

Ephedra sinica (Somlata/Ma Huang) and some other species of oriental *Ephedra* prove exceptional useful as bronchodilators. Original source of the alkaloid 1-ephedrine. The synthetic ephedrine is racemic, optically inactive because it has equal parts of dextro & levorotatory forms. The natural form has advantages as it is better tolerated. Ephedrine stimulates the sympathetic nervous system, relieving the bronchial spasm that underlies the asthmatic state, as well as other conditions that have a bronchospasm component such as emphysema. Allergic reactions respond well to *Ephedra* because of its action on the sympathetic nerves

Uses : The whole plant is used for medicine in the treatment of rhinitis, cold, fever, sinusitis, asthma and bronchitis.

Ephedra Tea : It is generally used in the form of

powder, decoction or tea. Pouring boiling water over a half teaspoonful of the powder and a half teaspoonful of leaves makes Somlata tea. To this liquor, sugar and milk can be added according to taste and given to the patient. To form the decoction one teaspoonful of powder is added to a cup of water, boiled and reduced to one-fourth its volume. The decoction is then strained and the residue is discarded. The decoction is used as medicine. The semisolid paste can be converted into 250 mg pills.

Dose :

Powder : Half a teaspoonful three times a day mixed with honey.

Decoction: 30 ml, three times a day with a little sugar.

Pills: Two pills three times a day with any hot drink. (500 mg.)

Haritaki (Terminalia Chebula)

The names of this herb is different languages are:

English	:	Black myrobalan
French	:	Myrobalana chebula
German	:	Rispiger
Hindi	:	Harara
Italian	:	Mirobalano nero
Arabic	:	Shagar

Properties

Taste	:	Five tastes
Quality	:	Dry and light
Virility	:	Hot
Post-assimilative effect	:	Sweet

Haritaki is a tree that grows upto 24-30 m in height. The leaves are 7.5 x 10 cm with sharp tips. The fruits are 1.5 - 3 cm long with five ridges on the outer side. The ripe fruit is dark brown in colour. The fruit pulp is used in medicine.

Uses : Haritaki is widely used as a tonic and as a laxative. It is beneficial in asthma, bronchitis, tonsillitis, laryngitis and pharyngitis. It is used in the treatment of piles, oedema, skin diseases, diarrhoea and eye diseases.

As a tonic for the prevention of asthma and other diseases, the powder or pulp of these fruits is given along with other materials, depending upon the season.

In the rainy season, its powder is given along with rock salt, in autumn with sugar, in winters with dry ginger powder, in spring with honey and in summer with jaggery. Generally, one teaspoonful of haritaki powder is given along with one teaspoonful of the Anupanas (adjuvant).

The powder of this fruit should be given at bedtime along with one-fourth quantity of rock salt in chronic bronchitis and asthma patients. The mixture of three drugs, namely, Haritaki (Terminalia chebula), Vibhitaki (Terminalia belerica) and Amalaki (Emblica officinalis) in equal quantities is called triphala. It should be given to the patients at bedtime in doses of one to two teaspoonfuls along with warm milk or water.

If bronchitis, asthma and cough are associated with constipation and malfunction of the liver, it should be given in the form of a decoction. The decoction is prepared by adding two teaspoonful of triphala powder to two ounces (1 ounce = 28.35 gm) of water and boiling. Reduce the mixture to one-fourth its initial volume. Thereafter, it should be strained through a cloth and given to the patient. As linctus, it is given to the patient twice a day with honey or warm milk. The common name of linctus is Agastya haritaki or Agastya rasayana.

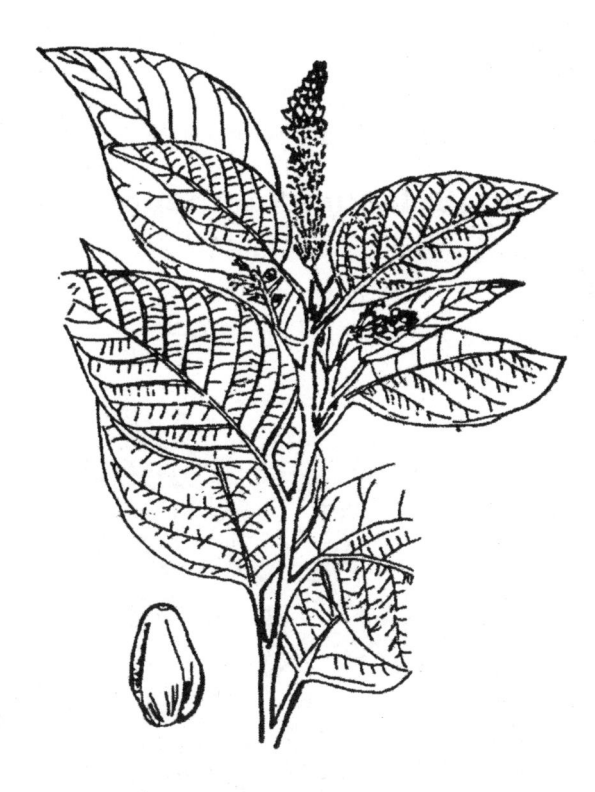

Haritaki (Terminalia chebula)

Abhayarishta

Along with a few other drugs, haritaki is kept in a jar, in which fermentation is allowed to take place. The alcoholic preparation obtained is very effective in piles, cough and asthma.

Dose :

Powder: Half to one teaspoonful, twice a day with warm water.

Decoction: 30 ml, twice a day with sugar on an empty stomach.

Linctus: 1-2 teaspoonfuls, 2-3 times a day with honey or warm milk.

Alcoholic Preparation: 30 ml twice a day after food with an equal quantity of water.

Kantakari (Solanum Xanthocarpum)

The names of this herb in different languages are:

English : Yellow berried nightshade
Italian : Bondue, Niceheri

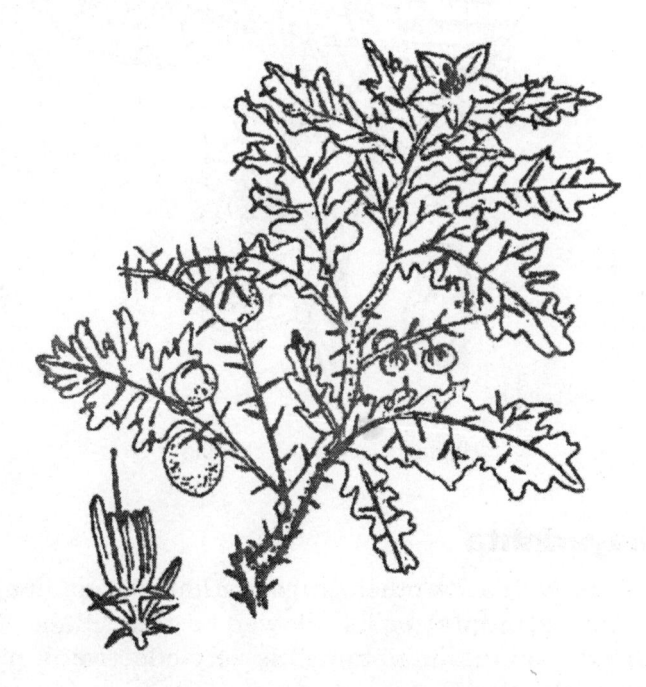

Kantakari (Solanum xanthocarpum)

Arabic : Badankare

Persian : Badanaganedashti

Properties

Taste : Bitter, Pungent

Quality : Light, Dry

Virility : Hot

Post-assimilative effect : Pungent

It is a thorny, herbal plant growing upto 30 cm - 1.2 m in height. The flowers are generally blue or white. The leaves are oval with irregular margins and have thorns on their back. Flowers and fruits appear in summer. Fruits are round, like small brinjals and yellow when ripe. The whole plant is used in medicine.

Uses : Kantakari is widely used in the treatment of bronchial asthma, cough and bronchitis. It is also beneficial in fever, sore throat, toothache, cold, vomiting and urinary tract infections. The whole plant is used in the form of powder or decoction.

Effect of Kantkari on Asthma : The beneficial effect of Kantkari on bronchial asthma has been validated scientifically. The effect is attributed to its property to deplete histamine from bronchial and lung tissue. Plant is also attributed with diuretic properties and hence used to increase urination.

Decoction : The decoction is prepared by boiling one tablespoonful of the powder with two cups of water, till it reduces to one-fourth of the initial volume. Then the liquid is strained. The residue is discarded. The liquid should be cooled and given to the patient with a little honey or jaggery to overcome its astringent taste.

Dose :

Decoction : 30 ml. three times a day

Powder : 2-3 g. three times a day with warm water.

Vasa (Adhatoda Vasaca)

The names of this herb in different languages are:

English : Malabar nut
French : Nayer de Malabar
Hindi : Arusa, Adalsa
Italian : Justicia arbonescente
Persian : Bansa
Arabic : Adhatudah

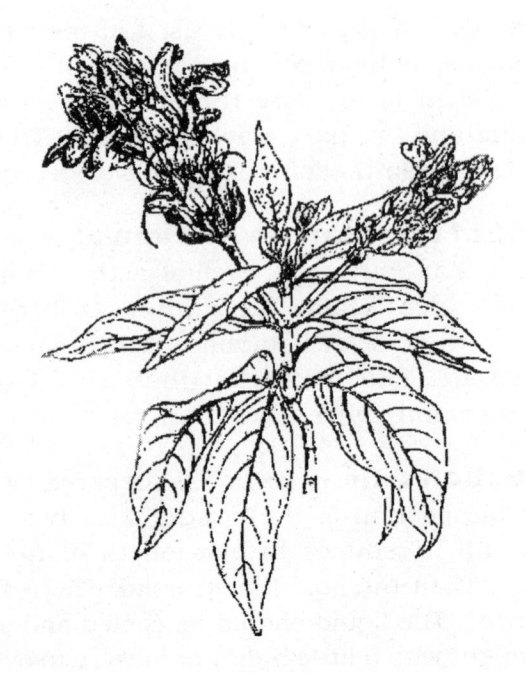

Vasa (Adhatoda vasaca)

Properties

Taste	:	Bitter and Astringent
Quality	:	Dry and Light
Virility	:	Cold
Post assimilative effect	:	Pungent

Action : *It alleviates Pitta & Kapha.*

It is small plant growing to a height of 1.2 -1.8 m. Flowers are white, violet or pink in colour. The petals are arranged in such a way that the flowers resemble the mouth of a lion. Therefore, it is called 'Simha mukhi' (simha – lion, mukhi – face). The leaves are broad, tapering towards the tip, smooth on the dorsum, slightly rough at the ventral side and yellowish – green in colour.

The entire plant is used in the medicine. Vasaka grows in the mountain and in hilly places.

Action on Nervous System : It causes depression of vagus nerve.

Action on Gastrointestinal System : Its stambhana action (due to its tastes viz. bitter and astringent) treats diarrhoea and dysentry especially dysentry with blood. It treats jaundice and fever of Kapha Pitta origin.

Action on Respiratory System : It acts as a good decongestant.

Adhatoda vasica extract with ginger, tulsi (holy basil), liquorice (Glycirhiza glabra) and honey treats persistent cough because it is an excellent mucolytic agent and treats asthma by relieving bronchospasm.

The bronchodilator action is comparatively less yet permanent.

The leaves are used in the treatment of respiratory

disorders in Ayurveda. Research performed over the last three decades revealed that the alkaloids, vasicine and vasicinone present in the leaves, possess respiratory stimulant activity. Vasicine, at low concentrations, induced bronchodilation and relaxation of the tracheal muscle. At high concentrations, vasicine offered significant protection against histamine induced bronchospasm in guinea pigs. Vasicinone, the auto-oxidation product of vasicine has been reported to cause bronchodilatory effects both *in vitro* and *in* vivo. In another study, vasicine showed appreciable bronchodilatory effect and marked respiratory stimulant activities whereas vasicinone showed relaxation of the tracheal muscle *in vitro* and bronchoconstriction *in vivo*. Of the two alkaloids, vasicinone was found to be more potent than vasicine, with potential anti-asthmatic activity comparable to that of disodium cromoglycate

The bronchodilatory effects of *Adhatoda vasica*. The alkaloids from this plant were found to offer pronounced protection against allergen-induced bronchial obstruction in guinea pigs when administered at the dosage of 10 mg/ml of aerosol.

Although the precise mechanism of action of the *Adhatoda vasica* alkaloids remains to be elucidated, these compounds are potentially useful phytochemicals in the management of allergic disorders and bronchial asthma. *Adhatoda vasica* is also accredited with antimicrobial properties with proven *in vitro* action against *Myco-bacterium tuberculosis* and reduction of gingival inflammation.

Uses : Vasaka is commonly used in the treatment of cough and asthma. It liquefies phlegm, helps in its removal from the chest and facilitates breathing. It is a bronchodilator, immuno-modulator and also an antimicrobial. It is also beneficial in piles (bleeding), jaundice, fever, tuberculosis, constipation and bleeding from different parts of the body.

Juice : The leaves of the plant are not juicey; therefore, some water has to be added while preparing the paste of juice.

Dose : One teaspoonful of Vasaka paste or juice three times a day with an equal quantity of honey or sugar.

Powder: The leaves should be dried in the shade before powdering because exposure to the sun while drying reduce its therapeutic efficacy.

Dose : 5 g three times a day.

To obtain better results in cough and asthmatic complaints, long pepper powder (2 g) or ginger powder (2 g) should be added to the powder or paste of Vasaka.

Decoction : The decoction is prepared by boiling one tablespoonful (15 g) of the powder with two cups of water till it reduces to one-fourth of its initial volume. Then the liquid is strained. The residue is discarded. The liquid should be cooled and given to the patient with a little honey. Because of its bitter taste, it might cause nausea. Therefore, a small quantity of honey may be added, as described above.

Dose : The decoction should be taken in a dose of one tablespoonful (15 ml) three times a day along with 1 teaspoonful (5 g) of sugar.

These preparations can be given safely to adults and children for long periods. Other preparations of vasaka are:

1. Vasavaleha
2. Vasa ghrta (Medicated ghee)
3. Vasarishta (Alcoholic preparations)

Pushkara Mula (Inula Racemosa)

The names of this herb in different languages are:

German	:	Blaweiris, Dentsche lisch
Persian	:	Gharsa
French	:	Lis sauvage, Flambe
Arabic	:	Rasan
English	:	Urris root
Hindi	:	Pohkaramula
Italian	:	Azurro, Iride ralvatica

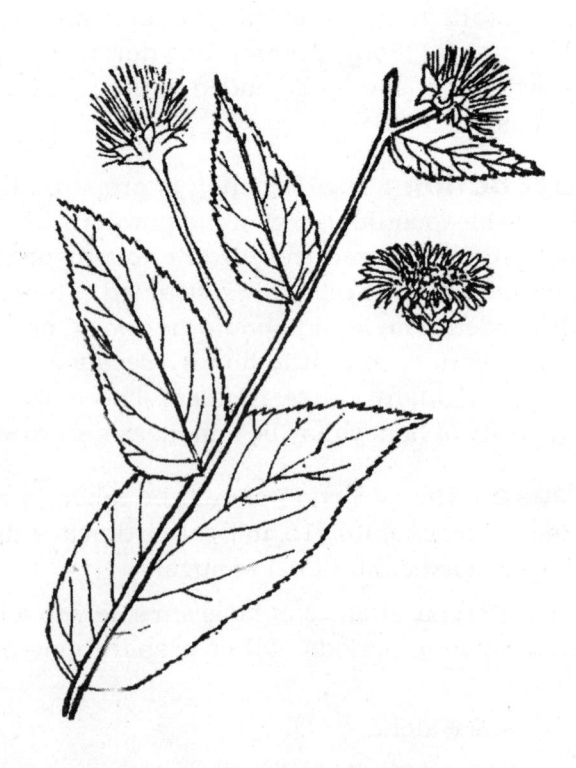

Pushkara Mula (Inula racemosa)

Properties

Taste	:	Bitter, Pungent
Quality	:	Light, Sharp
Virility	:	Hot
Post-assimilative effect	:	Pungent

Pushkara mula is an erect herbal plant growing to a height of 1-2 m. The flowers and fruits appear in autumn. It grows on the moist slopes of the Northern Himalays in the height of range of 2500-3000 m. It is also cultivated. The root is used for medicinal preprations. It possesses a characteristic penetrating odour.

Uses : Pushkara mula is used externally in the treatment of sprains and bruises. Internally, it is used in the treatment of cough, asthma, sore throat and pharyngitis.

Paste made from the root is applied externally for the treatment of bruises. The root of Pushkaramula is used internally in the form of powder or as tea.

Dose : One gram of the powder three times a day. To brew it as tea, half a teaspoonful (2.5 g) of the powder is added to a cup of water (with milk and sugar to taste) and given to the patient three times a day.

Management of Tamaka Shvasa (Bronchial Asthma) with Pushkarmooladi Choorna :

Bronchial asthma is recognized as primarily an inflammatory disorder leading to bronchospasm and microvascular leakage. There is a great role of immune system in pathogenesis of asthma. Charaka has given three drugs Sati, Pushkar, Amalaki combination in shwasa chikitsa. (Charaka Chikitsa 17/129).

This combination acts as anti-inflammatory, bronchodilator and immunomodulator. Shati (Hedychium spicatium) acts as an anti inflammatory, Pushkar acts as a bronchodialator, and Amalaki acts as a immunomodulator.

The equal parts of rhizome of Shati, roots of pushkarmool, and fruit of Amalaki after removing the seeds were fine powdered. Nine gram of the powder should be given in 3 divided doses with honey.

Pippali (Piper Longum)

The names of this herbal plant in different languages are:

Greek : Peperimakron
Hindi : Pipal, Piper

Pippali (Piper longum)

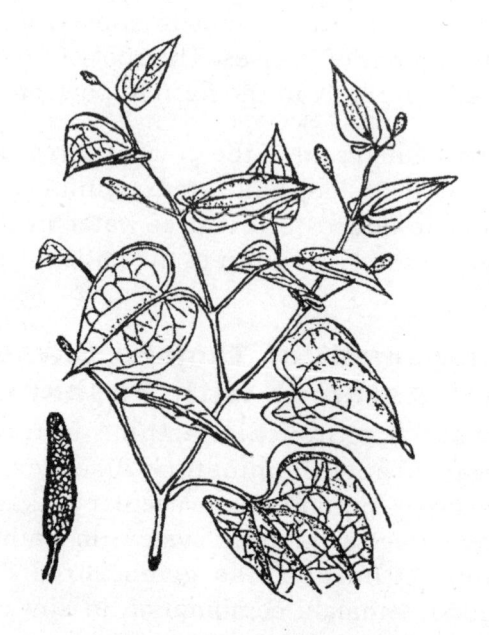

Arabic	:	Darjifil
German	:	Langer Pfeffer
English	:	Long pepper
French	:	Poivre long
Persian	:	Pilpil
Urdu	:	Pipul

Properties

Taste	:	Sweet (when fresh and wet), Pungent (dried)
Quality	:	Light, Sharp, Unctuous
Virility	:	Semi-hot
Post-assimilative effect	:	Pungent

Pippali is an aromatic climber with perennial woody roots. Fruit are ovoid; yellowish orange (brownish black when dry). Its root called pippali mula is also used as medicine. Pippali grows in nature in the mountain valleys and coastal areas of tropical regions. It is also cultivated in tropical and subtropical areas. The fruits and the root are used for medicine.

Piper longum (long pepper) has been used in Ayurveda in various formulations as an appetite stimulant, anticolic, antitussive and immunostimulant. The fruits contain 1% volatile oil, resin, alkaloids, piperine and piperlongumine and a terpenoid substance. The roots contain piperine, piperlongumine or piplartine. Isolation of Dihydrostigmasterol has also been reported.

The antiallergic activity of *Piper longum* has been studied. *Piper longum* extract effectively reduce passive cutaneous anaphylaxis against antigen-induced bronchospasm. In an *in vitro* study, a 30% protection of mast cells was observed.

In Ayurveda, the fruit has been used in the prevention of recurrent attacks of bronchial asthma. In a classic study, 240 children with asthma were subjected to long-term treatment with the fruit. 58.3% showed decreased severity of attacks. In another investigation, 20 children were studied for one year with the same treatment. Of these, 11 had no recurrence of attacks. All patients had a strongly positive skin test, which became negative in six and decreased significantly in 12 after five weeks of treatment.

Uses : Pippali is very useful drug. It is widely used in the treatment of cough, cold, asthma, tonsillitis, eosinophilia, pharyngitis, nausea, gout, epilepsy, colic, diseases of the liver and spleen, sleeplessness, anxiety and tuberculosis.

Powder or Paste : The dry powder is obtained by grinding the dry fruit. This powder is dissolved in some water to make a paste. The recomm-ended dose is 5 g three times a day. Sugar and milk can be added according to taste. It is also used in the form of decoction or tea. It is pungent in taste. Therefore, a little jaggery, sugar or honey is added to make it palatable.

It is also boiled with milk or added to ordinary tea. For headache and sleeplessness, the root is used in powder form; the dosage recommended is 5 g three times a day. In the form of tea one cup should be taken three times a day.

Pippali Rasayana : Pippali Rasayana is used for rejuvenating the body, especially in patients suffering from chronic asthma with emphysema, bronchiectasis and tuberculosis. Several approaches are adopted by the physician in the practice of rejuvenation therapy with this drug. In rejuvenation therapy, the smaller variety of pippali is more effective. Five fruits of long pepper are administered on the first day. Thereafter, the quantity is increased by five fruits per day till the tenth day. Then it is reduced by five fruits per day for the next 10 days. The course of treatment is usually for 20 days by which time the patient has consumed 500 fruits. The fruits of pippali should be taken in powder form and administered with honey or milk.

Anantmula
(Tylophora Indica, T. Asthmatica)

Sanskrit name : Anantamula

Common name : Indian ipecac

Properties

Taste	:	Bitter, Astringent
Quality	:	Dry, Light
Virility	:	Hot
Post-assimilative effect	:	Pungent

Parts used and where grown : Tylophora is a perennial, dark copper colored creeper native to the plains, forests, and hills of Southern and Eastern India. The portions of the plant employed medicinally are the leaves and root.

Historical or traditional use : This plant has been traditionally utilised as a folk remedy in certain regions of India, not only in the treatment of bronchial asthma, but for bronchitis, rheumatism, and dermatitis. In the latter half of the 19th century, it was called Indian ipecacuahna, as the roots of the plant have often been employed as an effective substitute for ipecac; this use to induce vomiting led to tylophora's inclusion in the Bengal Pharmacopoeia of 1884.

Powder from the dried leaves, root powder, and

decoction of the leaves or infusion of the root bark have been used traditionally in the treatment of respiratory afflictions such as chronic bronchitis and asthma. In recent years, the leaves have been used in the treatment of bronchial asthma.

Tylophora has been used in connection with the following conditions : Preparations containing dried powdered plant material are beneficial for the treatment of bronchial asthma and tropical eosinophilia. It is also useful in hay fever and diarrhoea.

Active constituents : The primary ingredient in tylophora is the alkaloid tylophorine. Laboratory research has shown this isolated plant extract exerts a strong anti-inflammatory action. Moreover, scientists suspect that tylophorine is able to interfere with the action of mast cells, which are key components in the process of inflammation. Mast cells are specialized types of cells in the body that lie along blood vessels and are found primarily in the skin, airways of the lungs, and gastrointestinal tract. When they are triggered by an allergen, they release the chemical histamine, which in turn leads to a wide number of symptoms familiar to allergy and asthma sufferers, such as itchy eyes, runny nose, chest tightness, and even diarrhoea. Together, these latter facts support tylophora's traditional use as an anti-asthmatic and anti-allergic medication by Ayurvedic practitioners.

The historical and laboratory findings have been validated by several human clinical trials using differing preparations of tylophora. One such study randomly assigned 110 bronchial asthma patients to receive one tylophora leaf (150 mg of the leaf by weight) or comparable placebo to be chewed and swallowed daily in the early morning for six days. At the end of one week, 62% of the patients consuming the tylophora reported experiencing moderate to complete relief of their asthma symptoms compared to 28% in the placebo group. Moreover, when patients were switched from the placebo to the active group and vice versa, similar positive trends could be seen, with 50% of the tylophora group and 11% of the placebo group reporting symptomatic relief. In a follow-up study, the alcoholic extract of crude tylophora leaves in 1 gram of glucose had comparable effects to that of chewing the crude leaf, with 56% of the patients reporting moderate to complete improvement in asthmatic symptoms compared to 32% in the placebo group.

In another clinical trial, 30 patients with a diagnosis of bronchial asthma for at least two years were assigned at random to one of two treatment groups consisting of 15 individuals each. One group received either 350 mg of tylophora leaf powder or placebo daily in the first week. In comparison, a second group of asthmatics were given a similar amount of the leaf for seven days followed by an anti-asthmatic herbal preparations. Overall, results of the study showed the amount of oxygen in the lung (e.g. vital capacity) increased in those using the leaf but decreased in those using the placebo. In addition, those taking the herb had a notable night–time reduction in their symptoms of shortness of breath.

The anti-Asthmatic activity of the plant is attributed to the presence of phenanthro-indolizidine alkaloids. An alkaloid mixture (0.17%) has been isolated from the aerial parts of the plant.

Tylophorine, the major alkaloid, has been studied extensively. The presence of tylophorine in the roots of the plant was first described in 1891. Subsequently, two crystalline alkaloids tylophorine and tylophorinidine were isolated.

Tylophorine

The extract of the plant shows anti-anaphylactic effect and leucopenia. The lymphocytes and eosinophils were found to be markedly reduced. The extract also shows brief, nonspecific anti-spasmodic action. The utility of this plant in the treatment of bronchial asthma could be attributed to its action on cell-mediated immunity. The plant extracts produce muscle relaxant effect, antagonism of smooth muscle stimulants and immuno-suppressive effects.

Coleus Forskohlii

Coleus forskohlii belongs to the Natural Order Labiatae (Lamiaceae), a family of mints and lavenders. The plant is the only known natural source of the unique adenylate cyclase activating drug, forskolin. Forskolin helps to enhance the production of compounds that relax the bronchial muscle.

Forskolin activates adenylate cyclase

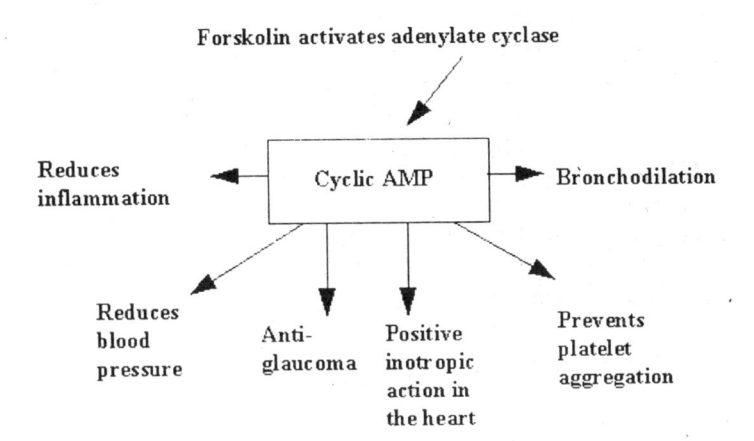

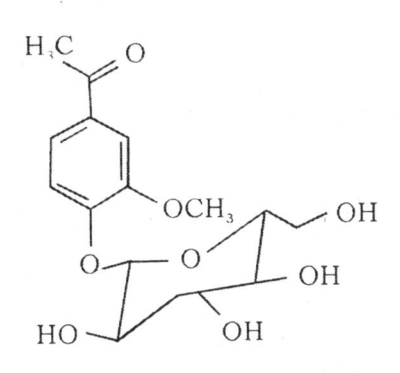

```
                    ┌───────────┐
Reduces      ←──────│ Cyclic AMP│──────→ Bronchodilation
inflammation        └───────────┘
```

Reduces blood pressure — Anti-glaucoma — Positive inotropic action in the heart — Prevents platelet aggregation

Androsin

Bharangi

Latin Name: Clerodendrum serratum.

Properties

Taste	:	Bitter, Astringent
Quality	:	Dry, Light
Virility	:	Hot
Post-assimilative effect	:	Pungent
Plant parts used	:	Roots, Leaves

Description : A shrub 0.9-2.4 m high, slightly woody, not very branched, stems bluntly quadrangular, young parts usually glabrous. It has pink white flower, numerous and striking.

Characteristics and Constituents : A sterolglucoside has been isolated. The root bark yields a glycosidic material, phenolic in nature. D-mannitol was isolated from the root bark with a yield of 10.9%. The powdered stem contains D-mannitol, ß-D glucoside of ß-sitosterol, ß-sitosterol and cetyl alcohol. From the bark the sapogenin mixture contains three major triterpenoid constituents – olconolic acid, queretaroic acid and serratagenic acid.

Actions and Uses : An aqueous extract produced a graded block of the responses to histamine on isolated guinea pig ileum. It blocked the histamine - induced contractions of the guinea pig tracheal chain preparations without affecting the response to acetylcholine. The saponin isolated from the rook bark caused a release of histamine from rat lung tissue. Continuous daily administration of the plant extract in the sensitised guinea pig causes a gradually developing protection against anaphylaxis. The anticholinestrase activity of the saponin was confirmed by acetylcholine responses on guinea pig tracheal chain preparation, isolated rat ileum and frog rectus muscles. The saponin also disrupted the rat peritoneal mast cells and blocked the effect of horse serum antigen.

A decoction of roots is used in asthma and bronchitis. The leaves are applied in the form of poultice in skin suppurations. The drug is used in fever. It is also used in sinusitis. It is recommended in inflammations of the eye.

In the doses used, no adverse reactions have been reported in man. Larger doses are reactive.

9

THINGS TO BE OBSERVED

COUGH AND ASTHMA

Cough is one of the most useful differences between asthma from allergens and asthma from infections. In allergic asthma cough is usually very mild, maybe absent, early in the attack. But towards the end of the attack it gets worse until the asthmatic starts coughing up mucus. Then the attack begin to get better and soon the shortness of breath ends. It should be easy to remember and be comforted by the quotation: "The allergic asthmatic coughs himself out of an attack."

In infectious asthma, cough usually start hours before, often one to three days before, and occasionally a week or more before the wheezing and shortness of breath. The cough is often severe and exhausting all during the attack. Cough continues after the attack is over and until the infection is cured. The doctor will know that the asthma will probably become severe and that the infection must be treated promptly when he is remind that: "The infected asthmatic coughs himself into an attack."

SPUTUM AND ASTHMA

Sputum can be quite a problem. When attacks of asthma get worse, the sputum gets sticker, drier, thicker, and harder to cough up. This starts what can be called a vicious circle. The more and stickier the sputum, the harder the cough and the harder the cough, the worse the asthma becomes.

In allergic asthma the sputum contains mucus, water, and some white blood cells. It is seldom a real problem if the attack is treated promptly. It can become a major problem if treatment is delayed and, particularly, if the asthmatic is breathing excessively dry air through his mouth, and if he doesn't drink enough fluid to keep his lung lining moist. In allergic asthma, hay fever is often present also. If there are any discharges from the nose, they too contain mucus, water, and some white blood cells. Sticky or wet, clear mucus from the nose is pretty reliable evidence that the asthma is allergic.

Infectious asthma can start in two ways: as a cold in the head or an infection in the lungs of people who are already asthmatics. A cold in the head can do either or both of two things in an asthmatic: It can cause sinus infection (sinusitis), or it can cause bronchitis. In either case, infectious asthma is the usual result.

Severity of Asthma

If he isn't wheezing, it isn't asthma. Second, you can get a pretty good idea of how severe the asthma is by looking at several things; the flesh above the collar bone, the muscles of the neck, the motions of the head, the spaces between the ribs and the size of the chest. How much longer does it take to get his breath out than in? Does he breathe in or out through his mouth or nose? What do these things mean? Why bother to look for them?

The flesh above the collarbone does not move in normal quiet breathing or in mild attacks. When asthma is troublesome, this flesh tends to bulge up a little when breathing out and sinks down when breathing in. In general, the more this flesh moves the more severe the asthma is.

The side muscles of the neck don't tighten or stand

out during quiet breathing or during an attack when he (or she) is breathing out. But they do tighten and stand out when he has to struggle to get a deep breath in. The muscles to look at start under the jaw on both side and end along the upper border of the ribs, just behind the collarbones. The hard the struggle to breathe in, the easier it is to see those muscles. The tightening of those muscles is easier to see than movements of the neck flesh in a fat people.

Certain movements of the head in order to breathe, during an attack, mean serious asthma. The head moves backwards and the chin upwards when it is hard to take in a quick deep breath. The head moves back to its usual position, or a little forward, during the longer efforts to get the breathe out. The more the head moves the more severe the attack of asthma, as a rule.

Changes in the spaces between the ribs and the size of the chest vary:

1. With the effort to breathe.
2. With the ability to breathe out all of the air breathed in with each breath.

During normal breathing the spaces between the ribs narrow slightly when breathing out and widen when breathing in.

The chest gets wider from side to side and thicker from front to back when breathing in. This is seen more easily in the lower rib and the breastbone areas from the side and from the front.

The striking thing in severe asthma is that all of the breath taken in (inhaled) can't quiet be breathed out (exhaled). The result in that, if the attack is not relived, the chest begins to look like a breath had just been taken in, when actually the breath had just been exhaled (breathed out). In such a case, the spaces between the ribs are wider and the front ribs are higher and further forward than before the attack. The size and shape of chest return to normal when the attack is over unless asthma has been frequent and severe for many years.

How much longer does it take to get air out than in? A healthy person breathes about 16 times a minute at rest. During each minute he breathes in about 24 seconds and breathes out about 36 seconds. This doesn't change much when he exercises moderately, although his breathing may be deeper. During a spell of asthma it takes longer to breathe out, so inhaling the air must be quicker. Using the second hand on your watch or clock, you can get some idea about how severe the asthma is by counting the number of seconds it takes: (a) to exhale ten times and (b) then count the number of seconds for ten inhalations. If the number of seconds spent breathing out is more than twice the number of seconds it takes to breathe in, the attack is either severe or is apt to become so.

Does he breathe in or out through his nose or mouth? A lot depends on whether the nose is clear or stuffy. If the nose is clear, air is usually inhaled and exhaled through the nose is mild attacks. When an attack becomes severe, the asthmatic usually breathes in through the mouth and out through the nose.

It is easy to tell when the nose is stuffy or clear. Simply press a finger on one side of the nose at a time, during four or five the stuffed side is closed. But if finger pressure closes the clear side, he quickly starts breathing through his mouth. This is called the "sniff test". When both sides of the nose are stuffy, he obviously has to breathe in and out through his mouth.

10

SARS

SEVERE ACUTE RESPIRATORY SYNDROME

Severe acute respiratory syndrome (SARS) is a respiratory illness that has recently been reported in Asia, North America, and Europe. The symptoms are somewhat like Pneumonia but not exactly. Pneumonia is a serious infection or inflammation of your lungs. The air sacs in the lungs fill with pus and other liquids. Oxygen has trouble reaching your blood. If there is too little oxygen in your blood, your body cells can't work properly. Because of this and spreading infection through the body pneumonia can cause death.

In 2000, pneumonia and influenza combined ranked as the seventh leading cause of death.

Pneumonia affects your lungs in two ways. Lobar pneumonia affects a section (lobe) of a lung. Bronchial pneumonia (or bronchopneumonia) affects patches throughout both lungs. Recently this disease which has been termed as SARS is spreading epidemically was considered initially as Pneumonia but as the symptoms were more grave and were not getting treated with the line of management of Pneumonia it is categorized as separate syndrome related to the Respiratory diseases.

SARS is caused by a virus known as coronavirus.

Coronaviruses are a group of viruses that have the

corona shape. These viruses cause respiratory illness such as cough, shortness of breath, etc. in humans. These viruses also cause respiratory, gastrointestinal, liver and neurologic disease in animals.

Symptoms of SARS

In general, SARS begins with a fever greater than 100.4 °F [>38.0 °C]. Other symptoms may include headache, an overall feeling of discomfort, and body aches. Some people also experience mild respiratory symptoms. After 2 to 7 days, SARS patients may develop a dry cough and have trouble breathing.

How SARS spreads

The primary way that SARS appears to spread is by close person-to-person contact. Most cases of SARS have involved people who cared for or lived with someone with SARS, or had direct contact with infectious material (for example, respiratory secretions) from a person who has SARS. Potential ways in which SARS can be spread include touching the skin of other people or objects that are contaminated with infectious droplets and then touching your eye(s), nose, or mouth. This can happen when someone who is sick with SARS coughs or sneezes droplets onto themselves, other people, or nearby surfaces. It also is possible that SARS can be spread more broadly through the air or by other ways that are currently not known.

Who is at risk for SARS

Most of the U.S. cases of SARS have occurred among travelers returning to the United States from other parts of the world with SARS. There have been very few cases as a result of spread to close contacts such as family members and health care workers. Currently, there is no evidence that SARS is spreading more widely in the community in the United States.

Clinical Criteria

- Asymptomatic or mild respiratory illness
- Moderate respiratory illness
  (a) Temperature of >100.4 °F (>38 °C)*, and
  (b) One or more clinical findings of respiratory illness (e.g., cough, shortness of breath, difficulty breathing, or hypoxia).
- Severe respiratory illness
  (a) Temperature of >100.4° F (>38° C)*, and
  (b) One or more clinical findings of respiratory illness (e.g., cough, shortness of breath, difficulty breathing, or hypoxia), and
     (i) radiographic evidence of pneumonia, or
     (ii) respiratory distress syndrome, or
     (iii) autopsy findings consistent with pneumonia or respiratory distress syndrome without an identifiable cause

Epidemiologic Criteria

- Travel (including transit in an airport) within 10 days of onset of symptoms to an area with current or recently documented or suspected community transmission of SARS†, or
- Close contact within 10 days of onset of symptoms with a person known or suspected to have SARS infection.

Laboratory Criteria

- Confirmed
  (a) Detection of antibody to SARS-CoV in specimens obtained during acute illness or >21 days after illness onset, or
  (b) Detection of SARS-CoV RNA by RT-PCR

confirmed by a second PCR assay, by using a second aliquot of the specimen and a different set of PCR primers, or
(c) Isolation of SARS-CoV
- Negative
  (a) Absence of antibody to SARS-CoV in convalescent serum obtained >21 days after symptom onset
  (b) Undetermined: laboratory testing either not performed or incomplete

Case Classification
- *Probable case:* meets the clinical criteria for severe respiratory illness of unknown etiology with onset since February 1, 2003, and epidemiologic criteria; laboratory criteria confirmed, negative, or undetermined.
- *Suspect case:* meets the clinical criteria for moderate respiratory illness of unknown etiology with onset since February 1, 2003, and epide-miologic criteria; laboratory criteria confirmed, negative, or undetermined.

Update on cases and countries
As of today (20 May, 2003), a cumulative total of 7739 probable SARS cases and 611 deaths have been reported from 29 countries.

Stability of the SARS virus in the environment
WHO has today published additional data on the stability of the SARS virus on different environmental surfaces.

The data, which come from studies conducted by laboratories in the WHO network, indicate that the SARS virus in sterilized stool can survive for 36 hours on a plastered wall or a formica surface, for 72 hours on a plastic surface or stainless steel, and for 96 hours on a glass slide.

Some News

Sick Patient Gives Clues

Tuesday, March 18, 2003

A pneumonia patient believed to have spread a mysterious respiratory illness to dozens of hospital workers in Hong Kong traveled to mainland China before he became ill.

Dr. Leung Ping-chung, who has been working throughout the pneumonia outbreak at Hong Kong's hardest-hit hospital, told *The Associated Press* the patient believed to have spread the illness was a man aged in his 40s who had visited Hainan island and other parts of southern China.

Health authorities are trying to determine whether disease outbreaks in Hong Kong, Vietnam and elsewhere are linked to an illness in mainland China's southern Guangdong province that recently sickened 305 people and killed five.

Leung said the patient, who has not been identified by name, is "still very sick" in the hospital.

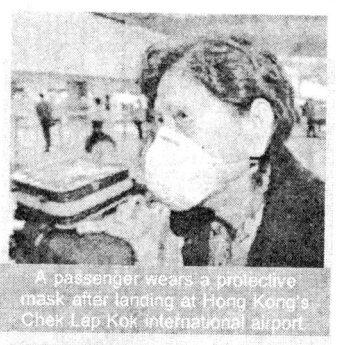

A passenger wears a protective mask after landing at Hong Kong's Chek Lap Kok international airport.

SYMPTOMS

The World Health Organization alerts travelers to be aware of the symptoms, which include:

People after February 1 with a history of fever greater than 100.4 °F (38 °C) *and* one or more respiratory symptoms including cough, shortness of breath, difficulty breathing and **one or more** of the following:

Close contact with a person who has been diagnosed with Severe Acute Respiratory Syndrome, or SARS. Close contact means having cared for, having lived with, or having had direct contact with respiratory secretions and body fluids of a person with SARS.

Recent history of travel to areas reporting cases of SARS.

He also criticized the territory's health authorities for allegedly playing down the threat posed by the disease.

"We must make sure and get prepared — something more serious may happen," said Leung, who works at the Prince of Wales Hospital and also is the chair professor of orthopedics at Hong Kong's Chinese University.

The university's medical school has close ties to the hospital, in suburban Shatin, and all of its medical professors have offices in the hospital.

On Monday, Hong Kong's health chief, Dr. Yeoh Eng-kiong, said that officials have identified the "index patient" who apparently has spread the disease to 68 people, mainly medical workers, at the Prince of Wales Hospital, but declined to provide any details about the patient.

Who extends SARS travel warnings to Toronto

Wednesday, April 23, 2003

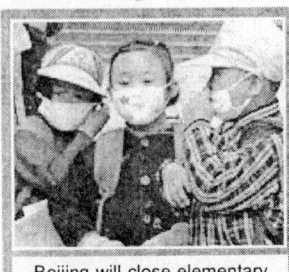

Canada criticizes action; Beijing closes schools

Atlanta, Georgia (CNN) — The World Health Organization stepped up its SARS-related travel warnings Wednesday, urging people to avoid unnecessary trips to China's Shanxi Province, Beijing and Toronto, Ontario.

Beijing will close elementary and secondary schools for two weeks as it intensifies efforts to contain SARS.

Canadian officials lashed out, saying the WHO advisory is an "overreaction" for their country. They plan to lodge a formal complaint to the WHO about the travel warning.

In Beijing — which has reported scores of new cases in recent days — the government said it would quarantine people suspected of having SARS and possibly infected buildings, according to Xinhua, China's official news agency. The WHO reports 2,305 confirmed cases in mainland China, including 106 deaths, and 1,458 cases in Hong Kong, with 105 deaths.

Also, city authorities announced that almost 2 million students will have their classes suspended for two weeks, starting Thursday in an effort to stem SARS.

In the advisory announcement, the WHO's David Heymann identified the three areas as having a "high magnitude of disease, a great risk of transmission locally outside the usual health workers ... and also there is exporting of cases."

"Today, one of the most important means of spreading diseases around the globe is air travel," said Heymann, executive director of the WHO's communicable diseases programs.

The advisory against nonessential travel to these areas will be in effect for three weeks. It is an extension of previous travel warnings to Hong Kong and China's Guangdong Province, where severe acute respiratory syndrome was first reported last year.

WHO has issued travel warnings because of illness in the past, warning travelers about plague in India in 1994.

With fears over the deadly illness taking grip, Chinese scientists have been mapping the genetic code from samples of the SARS virus in the hope of finding clues on treating and ultimately preventing it.

In doing so, they said, they have found considerable variations between samples taken in Beijing and those in Guangzhou, capital of Guangdong.

AYURVEDA VIEW

SARS as such if seen from an Ayurveda eye has some similarity with Shwasa roga though not exactly the same can be referred.

Doshas involved in the pathogenesis of SARS are mainly Prana Vayu and Udana Vayu along with Sadhaka Pitta and Avalambaka Kapha. Like in Shwasa Kapha obstructs the passage of Prana vayu and afflicts the Pranavaha srotas.

When this feature is observed along with fever we get the indication of "Antarvegi Jwara" according to Charaka Chikitsa 3/39 whereas the same if observed from Sushruta's point of view can be considered as "Gambhir Jwara"(Deep seated).

As in SARS the duration between the invasion of the pathogen and the manifestation of disease is not long; we consider this as the Agantuja jwara(Charaka nidana 1/30) or Bhutabhishangaj(Sushruta uttartantra 39/68) where the pathogen enters in the body and develops a disease or symptom and later the involvement of the doshas/dushyas and srotasa may convert it into a syndrome or in further complications.("Vyadheupri yo bhavet uttarkalja.......").

Here the invasion is of Cornovirus as bhuta.

Now as the pathogenesis is developing in a complicated manner it seems that it involves the doshas direct and also in overlapping manner i.e. Avaran.

- Kapha avritta prana vayu –Difficulty in breathing
- Udanavritta Apana vayu – Dyspnoea and cough.
- Pranavritta Udana vayu – Shirograha (Heaviness in head) and Pratishyaye (Rhinitis).

Prognosis

- Charaka says that Prana and Udana Vayu are the important doshas for body stability. As "Prana" is life and its Vikriti leads to Death. Similarly disturbance of Udana vayu causes loss of strength. [Charaka chikitsa sthana 28/234].

- Kapha Avritta Prana vayu is considered as very difficult to treat or incurable in Charaka Chi.28/233, which ultimately explains the incurability of SARS.

Herbs to boost upper respiratory tract immunity

Kalmegh : Andrographis panniculata.
- Rasa – Bitter;
- Guna – Light, Dry;
- Virya – Hot ;
- Vipaka – Pungent.

It is a useful antipyretic, anthelminthic, blood purifier, anti-inflamatory and gepato protective. (Wealth of India).

In Scandinavia, andrographis has been used as a treatment for colds. Reasonably good evidence tells us that it can reduce the severity of cold symptoms. It may also help prevent colds. Andrographis has been used to treat a wide range of parasites and microbial infections. The herb is also credited with stopping the spread of influenza in India during the 1919 epidemic. However, laboratory studies have shown no direct biocidal activity on bacteria such as *Staphylococcus pseudomonas* and coliform species. Laboratory investigations with a purifed andrographis compound have shown no effects against the HIV virus. It is now thought that the mode of action of andrographis is via an effect on the immune response rather than specific antimicrobial activity. This effect on immune response is thought to be mediated via the adrenal glands.

Shati : Hedychium spicatum. It is perennial shrub.

- Rasa – Pungent, Bitter, Astringent;
- Guna – Light, Sharp;
- Virya – Hot;
- Vipaka – Pungent.

It pacifies vata – kapha.

It is an appetizer, analgesic, digestive. It is useful in anorexia, cough, cold, asthma, hiccups, diseases of blood and pyrexia. (Dhanwantri nighantu)

Part used – Tubers. In the form of powder 1-3 gm.

Vanapsha : Viola odorata.

- Rasa – Sweet, Bitter;
- Guna – Light, Dry;
- Virya – Cold;
- Vipaka – sweet.

It pacifies vata and pitta and expectorates kapha.

Decoction of whole plant is used in cold, cough and bronchitis. It's anti microbial, analgesic, anti pyretic and anti inflammatory.

Dosage : 3-6gm in the form of decoction.

Yashtimadhu : Glycerrhiza glabra.

- Rasa – sweet;
- Guna – Heavy and unctuous;
- Virya – Cold;
- Vipaka – Sweet.

It is one of the best vitalizing herb. It enhances the energy level quickly when its fine powder is taken along with ghee. In tubercular cough fine powder of Yashti-madhu and Sitopaladi churna in 2:1 proportion to be licked with honey and ghee relieves the phlegm.

It nurtures all seven dhatus hence works well as a rasayana, boosts ojus formation.

Usnea : The herb's use dates back to ancient China where it was called Sunlo and was used to cool an overheated system and treat surface infections Usnea is a lichen — part fungus, part algae Usnic acid and its derivatives appear to be the main active constituents in *Usnea spp.* Usnic acid is believed to work against gram-positive bacteria by disrupting cell functions and thereby preventing adenosine triphosphate (ATP) formation and oxidative phosphorylation. Human cells are less permeable to usnic acid and so are not adversely affected.[1]

Elderberry Sambucus Spp. : Investigations also show that elderberry anthocyanins enhance immune function by boosting the production of cytokines.[2] These unique proteins act as messengers in the immune system to help regulate immune response, thus helping to defend the body against disease. An oftcited Israeli study on the anti-viral activity of elderberry extract found that in vitro elderberry extract reduced hemagglutination of red blood cells and inhibited replication of a number of strains of influenza A and B in cell cultures. In the same paper, administration of elderberry extract to 27 patients with influenza shortened the duration of flu symptoms. In a Swiss study, elderberry extract inhibited replication of avian influenza virus in a human breast cancer cell line.[3] And in vitro studies conducted by the Southern Research Institute using elderberry extracts from Artemis International showed inhibition of herpes virus in cell cultures.[4]

Woad Leaf Da qing ye : It kills some kinds of bacteria, including some strains resistant to sulfa drugs. In humans, indican is reportedly anti-bacterial, and will reduce fevers and swellings, and fight skin infections. Actions of Woad Leaf, Isatis, broad spectrum anti-bacterial, anti-inflammatory, detoxicant.

Reishi ganoderma lucidum : Reishi is particularly beneficial for individuals with asthma and other respiratory complaints. It has a healing effect on the lungs. "Reishi is good for respiratory strength and for coughing." At least one population study confirms this claim. When more the 2000 Chinese with chronic bronchitis took reishi syrup during the 1970s, within two weeks, 60 to 90% felt better and reported an improved appetite, according to "Medicinal mushrooms," by Christopher Hobbs, published in *Herbs for Health*, Jan/Feb 97.

Other herbs : Tulsi, Pippali, Gaujawan, Khatmi, Khoobkalan, Kooth, Lavanga, Shunthi etc.

GLOSSARY OF TERMS

Abhishyandi: Tendency to obstruct or block the channels of circulation.

Agni: Fire, that completes different body metabolism.

Alochaka: A variety of pitta which is located in the eyes and controls the function of eyes – vision.

Ama: Undigested macromolecules of food which form toxin.

Amlavetasa: Citrus fruit (variety of lemon).

Anuloman: Downward movement of vata.

Anaha: Distention of abdomen due to wind formation in stomach.

Anila: Synonym of vata.

Anupana: Vehicle or adjunct for drug administration.

Arishta: An alcoholic drink prepared by fermentation.

Asana (s): Third step of 'hatha yoga' involving the practice of physical postures.

Asava: Like arishta, it is also an alcoholic preparation prepared by fermentation.

Avran: Covering or overlapping of one dosha over another thereby reflecting the symptoms of one that covers & minimizing the signs of being covered.

Basti: Medicated enema.

Bhasma: Powder of a substance obtained by calcination.

Bodhaka: A variety of Kapha located on the tongue.

Churna: Powder.

Dhatvagni: (Metabolic enzymes) result in formation of seven dhatus.

Dhauti: One of the six purificatory measures of yoga.

Dhyana: Seventh step among eight steps of hatha yoga – meditation.

Doshas: Factors responsible for controlling physiological activities of the body, three in number, namely; Vata, Pitta & Kapha.

Ghrta: Medicated ghee.

Haritaki: Name of a medicinal plant; botanical name, *Terminalia chebula.*

Hingu: Ferula narthex

Hridya rog: Diseases related to heart.

Kala Namak: Black salt/ Rock salt.

Kalimirch: Black pepper.

Kalpa: A therapy which is used for rejuvenation of the body.

Kapha: One of the three dosas, serving as a lubricant of the tissue elements among other functions.

Khavaigunya: The impairment of the functional integrity of the channels, leading to its inability to perform its normal functions. (Kha= space).

Kumbhaka: Second stage of Pranyama i.e. Retention of breath.

Kvatha: Decoction, toe.

Lauha: Iron preparations.

Leha: Linctus.

Madhucchista: Bee wax.

Maruta: Synonym of vata.

Matulunga : Citrus fruit (variety of lemon).

Mudras & Bandhas: Postures and locks in yoga procedures.

Nasya: Use of oil, Ghrita or some other medication through nostrils.

Neti: One of the six pacificatory measures in yoga.

Pachakagni: Digestive fire.

Pandu: Deficiency of Hb - Anaemia.

Peya: Thin gruel (cereals with 14 parts water).

Phanta: Hot infusion.

Pilu: Salvadora persica.

Pippali: Name of a medicinal plant; botanical name, *Piper longum*.

Pishti: This is prepared by triturating the drug with the specified liquids and exposing to sun or moonlight.

Pitta Sthan: Site in the body where *Pitta dosha* is found.

Pranayam: Breath - controlling exercises.

Puraka: First stage of Pranyama i.e. inhalation of breath.

Rajyakshama: Tuberculois.

Rasa Kalpa: Preparations, which have metallic & mercury contents.

Rasayan: Rejuvenation/ Immunity enhancer.

Rechak: Third stage of Pranayama i.e. exhalation/ release of breath.

Sadhaka Pitta: One of the five varieties of pitta located in the heart region.

Samadhi: One of the eight steps of hatha yoga entering into deep meditation.

Sapta Dhatu: Seven fundamental body tissues.

Sarjaras: Resin of Shorea robusta.

Sattvika: Adjective of sattva-food which promotes noble qualities in a person.

Shatkarmas: Six eliminative or cleansing techniques of Yogic therapy.

Shunthi: Dry ginger powder.

Srotas: Micro and Macro channels.

Srotodushti: Vitiation of channel (Srota).

Stambhana: Astringent.

Tamas: One of mansik dosha or attribute.

Tridoshaja: Diseases caused by aggravation of all the three doshas.

Udavarta: Upward movement of wind in stomach.

Ujjai, sheetali: Breathing through alternative nostrils.

Upnaha: Fomentation.

Utkarika : Warm medicated boluses.

Vaman: Cleansing through upper tract (Emesis).

Vasti: Use of medicaments by anal route as enema.

Vida: Type of salt.

Vimarggaman: The flow of the fluid, in the affected area, through channels other than its own.

Virechan: Cleansing through lower tract (Purgation).

Vyadhi: The condition that brings sorrow i.e. an ailment.

Yogavahi: A therapeutic quality of a drug carrying the properties of the other drug mixed or boiled with it.

ABBREVIATIONS

PNS	Para Nasal Sinuses
O_2	Oxygen
CO_2	Carbon Dioxide
ABG	Arterial Blood Gases
PO_2	Amount of Oxygen dissolved in Plasma
PCO_2	Amount of Carbon Dioxide dissolved in Blood
HCO_3	Bicarbonate
B.E.	Base Excess
$AaDO_2$	Alveolar / Arterial Oxygen
HVS	Hyperventilation Syndrome
GIT	Gastro Intestinal Tract
ECG	Electrocardiogram
COAD	Chronic Obstructive Airway Disease
AR	Allergic Rhinitis
IgE	Immunoglobulin E
URT	Upper Respiratory Tract
LRT	Lower Respiratory Tract
APGAR	Air entery, Grunting, Respiration
COPD	Chronic Obstructive Pulmonary Disease
ROAD	Reversible Obstructive Response Disease

EAR	Early Asthmatic Response
LAR	Late Asthmatic Response
BHR	Bronchial Hyperreactivity
REM	Rapid Eye Movement (Type of sleep)
FEV_1	Forcefully Expired Volume (in the first second of FVF)
ECT	Electro Therapy (Kind of shock therapy)
SARS	Severe Acute Respiratory Syndrome

BIBLIOGRAPHY

AGHARKAR, S.P. 1953, Gazzette of Bombay State, General-A, Botany Pt. I - Medicinal Plants, Bombay.

AINSLIE, WHITELAW. 1826, Materia Medica Vol. I & II, Longman Press.

ANCIENT SCIENCE OF LIFE Vol. III No. 3 Jan.

ARYA VAIDYA SALA. 1995, Indian Medicinal Plants Vol. I, II, III, IV, Orient Longman, Hyderabad.

ASHTANG HRIDYA, Motilal Banarasi Das, New Delhi.

ASHTANG SAMGRAHA with Hindi commentry, Vol. I, Gupta A Krishndas Academy, 1993, Varanasi, Ist ed. Reprint.

AYURVEDIC MATERIA MEDICA, H.V. Savnur, Sri Satguru pub. India 1988.

AYURVEDIYE KRIYA SHARIR, Desai Ranjit Rai, Baidyanath Ayurved Bhawan, Nagpur, 7th ed. 1992.

BHANDARI, CHANDRARAJ 1951-57, Vanoushadhi Chandrodya, 10, Parts. Hindi, Varanasi.

BHAVA PRAKASHA of Sri Bhavamishra Edited with Vidyothini Hindi Commentory — Pandit Sir Brahma Shankar Mishra.

BHELA : BHEL SAMHITA - C.C.R.I.M.H. Pub. 31, New Delhi, 1977.

BHAVAPRAKASH NIGHANTU with commentory by Bramha Shankar Shastri, Chaukhamba, Varanasi, 1984.

BHAVAPRAKASH NIGHANTU with commentory by Bramha Shankar Shastri, Chaukhamba, Varanasi, 1984.

CHARAKA SAMHITA, ENGLISH, Shree Gulab Kunverba Ayurvedic Society, Jamnagar. Vol. I-V, Ed. 1949.

CHARAKA SAMHITA with Ayurveda Dipika Commentary, Dr. Acharya Y.T., Part 1-2, Chaukhamba Sanskrit Samsthan, Varanasi, 4th Ed. 1994.

DHYANI, S.C. The Pharmacological Aspects of Ayurveda.

DRAVYA GUNA VIGYAN, Yadavji Trikamji Acharya, Chaukhamba, Varanasi.

DWARKANATH, C. Introduction to Kayachikitsa. Popular Book Depot, 1959.

HOBBS C. *Usnea :* The herbal antibiotic. Capitola (CA): Botanic Press; 1986. 9-13.

KRISHNAMURTHY K.H., Wealth of Sushruta, Jawaharlal Institute of Ayurveda, Coimbatore, 1991.

MEHTA A.K., SHARMA R.N. — HEALTH AND HARMONY THROUGH AYURVEDA, 2003.

NIGHNANTU ADARSHA, Vol. 1 & 2 By, Bapalal G. Vaidya, Chaukhamba Bharati Academy, Varanasi, 1968.

N.S.K. 1967, VACHASPATI KOSH – A Hindi-Latin Dictionary of Economic Plants Among Certain Adibasi in India, Bull Bot. Suv. India 15, Delhi.

SAUTER C, WOLFENSBERGER C. Anticancer Activities as well as Antiviral and Virus-enhancing Properties of Aqueous Fruit Extracts from Fifty-six European Plant Species. *Eur J Clin Oncology* 1989; 25(6) : 987-90.

SHARMA, R.K. and BHAGVAN DASH 1976, Charaka Samhita, Vol. 1 and 2, Chowkhamba Sanskrit Series, Varanasi, India.

The Student's SANSKRIT — ENGLISH DICTIONARY — Vaman Shivram Apte, Govt. of India, 1987.

TURPIN, J. et al. Antiviral evaluation of elderberry extracts and standardized powder. Southern Research Inst. Frederick, MD. Unpublished 2000.

WATZL B, ROLLER M, BARTH SW, RECHKEMMER G. Anthocyanines Stimulate Cytokine Production (TNF-Alpha, IL-2) in Human Mononuclear Cells. Paper presented at: International Workshop on Immunonutrition; June 24-25, 2000; at Schloss Rauischholzhausen, Austria.

INDEX

A

Abhisyandi 103

Abhrak 132

Acidity 21, 22, 113

Adhatoda vasica 106, 149, 150

Agantuja 174

Agastya haritaki 132, 145

Agni 44, 45, 72, 82, 83, 87, 125, 138

Agoraphobia 29, 187

Albiz malt 106, 127, 133

Allergens 7, 39, 41, 43, 48, 49, 53, 54, 55, 57, 62, 63, 71, 82, 128, 163

Alochaka 75, 179

Alveoli 14, 15, 19, 22, 23, 27, 42, 44, 46, 51, 83, 88, 120, 121, 139

Ama 80, 82, 83, 87, 97, 99, 102, 128, 179

Amniotic fluid 44, 45, 46, 47

Anaha 91, 179

Ancillary components 106

Annavaha srotas 82

Antarvegi jwara 174

Anti-catarrhals 106, 133

Anti-microbial 106, 133

Antigens 60, 63

Apana 74, 88, 174

Apgar 44, 183

Aptarpana 104
Arterial blood gases 21, 44, 183
Asana 112, 115, 179
Asthi 79, 81
Atopic 39, 40, 43, 50, 57, 63, 67, 84
Avran 8, 88, 179

B

Bacteriostatic 47
Banana 96, 100
Banapsha 106
Basti 92, 111, 179
Bharangi 8, 106, 130, 131, 133, 161
Bhrajaka 75
Bhutabhishangaj 174
Bodhaka 77, 179
Boswellia serrata 106, 135
Brain cortex 14
Bronchi 12, 15, 34, 57, 67, 68
Bronchial carcinoma 68
Bronchial tubes 38, 97, 103, 105, 139
Bronchiectasis 31, 34, 68, 139, 156
Bronchitis 9, 31, 32, 34, 40, 52, 58, 67, 93, 97, 105, 113, 121, 126, 127, 141, 142, 144, 147, 157, 158, 162, 164, 176, 178
Bronchodilator 27, 57, 67, 142, 149, 150, 154

C

Capillary bed 46
Cellular respiration 13, 14
Chain reaction 7, 48

Chywanprash 106
Clerodendrum serratum 106, 161
Clubbing 68
Coleus forskohlii 8, 106, 160
Conchae 11
Coronavirus 167
Cosmetics 7, 50
Cyanosis 58, 68

D

Dermatitis 43, 63, 67, 157
Dharana 112
Dhatu 7, 8, 72, 79, 80, 81, 85, 88, 182
Dhatvagni 83, 180
Dhauti 111, 180
Diaphragm 12, 14, 15, 16, 30, 45, 49, 114, 117, 118, 120, 121
Discontent 76
Draksharishtha 132

E

Elderberry sambucus 177
Envy 3, 76
Eosinophils 52, 55, 56, 57, 61, 62, 160
Epiglottis 12
Epithelial cells 52, 61
Expectorant 133, 137, 141

F

Foetal lungs 44
Formaldehyde 50

G

Gambhir jwara 174
Gas exchange 13, 14, 45
Gastric 73, 74
Gaujawan 178

H

Haridra khand 132
Haridradi churna 131
Haritaki 8, 98, 105, 126, 132, 133, 143, 144, 145
Histamine 63, 147, 150, 158, 162
Hooka 125
Hridya 180, 185
Hypertrophy 59
Hyperventilation 29, 30, 49, 183

I

Immunological 62
Infections 24, 32, 34, 39, 40, 47, 51, 53, 55, 58, 72, 106, 147, 163, 175, 177, 178
Influenza 31, 32, 33, 167, 175, 177
Irritants 34, 53, 58, 93

J

Jatamansi 107, 125

K

Kalmegh 175
Kantkari 147
Khatmi 178
Khavaigunya 82, 180
Khoobkalan 178

Kledaka 77
Kooth 178
Kunjala 111

L

Langhan 102
Lavang 178
Leukotriene 106
Long pepper 96, 100, 101, 105, 126, 131, 133, 141, 151, 155, 156

M

Macrophages 52, 56
Mahabhuta 44, 72
Majja 79, 81
Mamsa 79, 81
Mast cell 52, 55, 56, 57, 59, 60, 61, 64, 155, 158, 162
Meda 79
Metabolic acidosis 25, 26
Methacholine 63
Moti bhasma 132
Moti pishthi 132
Mudras 122, 181
Myocardial ischaemia 30

N

Narcotics 9, 14
Nauli 111
Negative pressure breathing 15
Nervous tension 53
Neti 111, 112, 181
Niyama 112

O

Ocimum Sanctum 123
Olfactory nerve 50, 116
Orthopnoea 66

P

Pachaka 75
Pachakagni 83, 181
Panchkarma 5, 128, 129
Pandu 181
Percussion 35, 68
Pickles 55, 100
Pippaladya lauha 132
Pleura 12, 46
Pneumonia 31, 33, 35, 167, 169, 171
PNS 183
Prana 45, 74, 80, 88, 116, 122, 130, 174, 175
Pranayama 111, 112, 115, 116, 119, 120, 121, 122
Pranic biodetector 115
Pranvaha srotas 81
Pratyahara 112
Praval pishthi 132
Pregnancy 7, 46, 47, 64, 95
Pulmonary volumes 16

R

Rages 97
Rajyakshma 35
Rakta 32, 33, 79, 81
Ranjaka 75
Rasa 79, 80, 81, 87, 131, 132, 140, 175, 176, 181

Raupya 132

Receptors 22, 48, 49, 60

Reishi 178

Relaxant 160

Residual volume 18

Respiratory acidosis 25

Rhinitis 31, 32, 43, 51, 62, 63, 67, 83, 92, 105, 142, 174, 183

Rhonchi 67, 68

Rock salt 96, 98, 123, 124, 126, 144, 180

S

Sadhaka 75, 174, 181

Samadhi 112, 181

Samana 74

Sankhpraksalana 111

Saponin 162

SARS 8, 167, 168, 169, 170, 171, 172, 173, 174, 175, 177, 184

Season 7, 53, 63, 64, 84, 101, 128, 140, 144

Shatayadi Churna 131

Shatkarma 122

Shleshaka 77

Shodhana 104, 123

Shringyadi churna 131

Shrung Bhasma 132

Shukra 79, 81

Shwas kaasa chintamani rasa 132

Shwas kuthar 132

Sinuses 11, 53, 106, 133, 183

Sinusitis 32, 39, 40, 127, 142, 162, 164

Sitopaladi churna 131, 176

Srotas 8, 80, 81, 82, 86, 87, 174, 182
Stress 30, 39, 41, 49, 58, 72, 85, 86, 99, 107, 116, 117, 118, 133
Sulfites 54, 55
Surfactant 42, 45, 46
Sympathetic 15, 94, 114, 125, 142

T

Tachycardia 67
Tarpaka 77
Tejovatyadya ghrita 132
Temptations 97
Tenacious mucus 87
Tidal volume 18, 66, 119
Tonsils 11, 33, 51
Trataka 111
Triggers 27, 41, 51, 133
Triphala 144
Tuberculosis 31, 35, 36, 83, 150, 156
Tulsi 106, 123, 133, 149, 178
Turmeric 100, 105, 126, 127, 139, 141
Tylophora indica 105, 157

U

Udana 74, 88, 174, 175
Ulcers 140
Urges 7, 32, 77, 78, 79, 82, 83, 92, 96, 98
Usnea 177, 186

V

Vacha 107, 133

Vanapsha 176
Viola odorata 106, 176
Vital capacity 18, 30, 120, 159
Vyadhi 8, 84, 182
Vyana 74

W

Wheat flour 101
Wheezing 34, 37, 38, 39, 57, 58, 64, 67, 163, 164
Woad leaf 177, 178

Y

Yama 112, 122
Yashtimadhu 106, 133, 176
Yoga kriyas 112
Yogasana 115